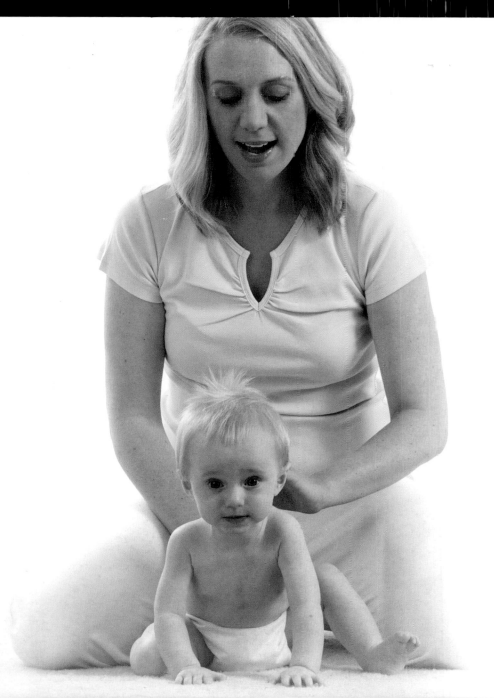

Developmental Baby Massage

THERAPEUTIC TOUCH TECHNIQUES FOR MAKING
YOUR BABY STRONGER, HEALTHIER, AND HAPPIER

PETER WALKER

FAIR WINDS
PRESS

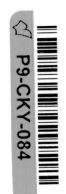

Text © 2000, 2009 Peter Walker

Illustrations and compilation © 2000, 2009 Carroll & Brown Publishers Limited

First published in the UK in 2009 by Carroll & Brown Publishers Limited

20 Lonsdale Road

Queen's Park

London NW6 6RD

First published in the USA in 2011 by

Fair Winds Press, a member of

Quayside Publishing Group

100 Cummings Center

Suite 406-L

Beverly, MA 01915-6101

www.fairwindspress.com

15 14 13 12 11   1 2 3 4 5

ISBN-13: 978-1-59233-483-4

ISBN-10: 1-59233-483-0

Digital edition published in 2011

eISBN-13: 978-1-61058-134-9

A CIP catalog record for this book is available from the British Library.

Managing Art Editor Emily Cook

Photography Jules Selmes

Printed and bound in China

Foreword

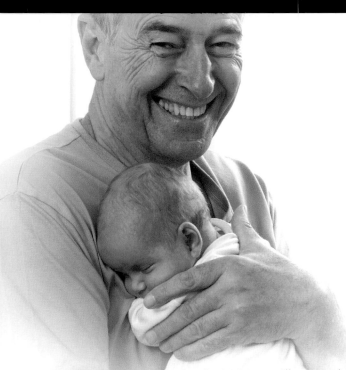

Since its first publication in 2000, my illustrated guide to developmental baby massage has introduced many thousands of parents to one of the most useful skills they can acquire. Through a parent's loving touch, babies receive many physical and emotional benefits. They relax and gain confidence and closeness with their parents and, as they develop, they lose the "physiological flexion" imposed by their position in the womb and start to gain a fuller range of movement.

Parents also benefit, as these techniques encourage loving attachment and more confidence in holding and handling, and can also be used to secure the full structural health and fitness of their baby.

This new edition has been fully revised and includes additional sequences that can be successfully used from birth onwards. It also features a spiral binding, enabling the book to be placed at eye level—on or alongside your massage surface—for easy and accessible, hands-free guidance.

The most powerful massage that your baby will ever receive during his lifetime is birth itself, which comes with the contractions of a vaginal delivery. During this time, the prolonged contractions of the uterus both pushed your baby through the birth canal and stimulated his peripheral nervous system and major organs in preparation for life outside the womb. By continuing a similar pattern of physical stimulation as your baby develops, you are following nature's way of boosting your baby's resilience. And, if your baby needed to be delivered by Caesarean section, this could prove to be even more necessary as he will not have had that early stimulation.

The techniques in this book are specifically devised to give you and your baby all the benefits of orthodox massage, while also helping your baby to fulfill his physical potential at each phase of development—from birth to sitting to standing and mobility. Acting on both the muscles and the joints, these techniques convey all the benefits of a loving touch and also ensure that your baby achieves full flexibility as he becomes mobile. Moreover, they ensure a level of relaxation that means that as your baby develops—both physically and emotionally—he is more likely to be "trauma free," maintain good posture and enjoy the self-confidence that accompanies a wide range of physical movement.

Developmental baby massage is highly therapeutic; both preventative and curative, it offers a form of immediate and convenient treatment. It can be used to alleviate stiff or floppy joints, wind, colic, constipation and other minor ailments and to bring an element of relief and assistance to children with additional needs. It also can enable you to uncover any potential physical problems.

How to use the book

- The book is designed to stand up on its own, so that you can refer to the text and leave your hands free to massage your baby.

- The top page of each exercise explains the purpose and the benefits of the massage, and the bottom page shows you how to do it, step by step.

- Boxed text highlights any contraindications or important issues to bear in mind while you massage your baby.

Developmental Baby Massage begins by introducing you to the physical and emotional benefits of massaging your child.

1 **Chapter one** shows you how to use touches and strokes—either with your baby dressed or undressed—in order to develop a close relationship with him in his first few weeks and to help him relax more fully and thrive.

2 **Chapter two** demonstrates an effective full-body massage routine along with everything you need to know—about the preparation, strokes, oils and ambience— needed to make it successful. Practiced regularly, this toe-to-top routine, along with the early touches, will promote emotional security and the prime physical attributes that constitute good posture, health and fitness. It will enable you to promote and maintain your baby's strength and suppleness. The techniques can also bring to light and alleviate any hidden areas of muscular tension and joint inflexibility.

3 **Chapter three** shows you how to use massage in later babyhood to help your baby to secure and maintain a healthy and comfortable sitting posture.

4 **Chapter four** keeps pace with your baby who, as he becomes more mobile, will want to explore his wide range of physical movement. This is the time to introduce some soft baby yoga, fun and games that engage your baby in versatile movement. These movements are designed to maintain existing suppleness and promote strength, balance and good posture while sitting and standing. At the end of this chapter you also can discover which time is best for you to massage your mobile baby.

5 **Chapter five** covers some common complaints and shows how massage and movement can be used to prevent and alleviate these conditions. Additional needs are also discussed, and there is advice on how massage can complement existing forms of treatment and therapy.

Contents

The Benefits of Touch

Touch is the newborn's first language—it is her prime means of communication and plays an essential role in the forming of early parent–child relationships. Massaging your baby allows you to express emotional affection and to fulfill your baby's need for physical contact. The benefits of massage are both emotional and physical, so your baby will achieve all-round wellbeing.

Emotional

With every emotional change there is a muscular reaction. By easing muscular tension, baby massage calms the emotions and helps to relieve some of the trauma and anxiety associated with birth and a new environment, and later on, with weaning. There is also a variety of other emotional benefits. Massaging your baby:

- Introduces a unique level of confidence and trust to your relationship.
- Brings fathers more in touch with their babies—giving them the opportunity to strengthen their relationship and learn how to handle their babies with confidence.
- Reduces the circulation of cortisol—a stress hormone in the bloodstream—if done regularly. This reduction is constant and maintained between massage sessions.

- Stimulates the release of the body's natural opiates—endorphins—which subdue pain. Together with the reduction of cortisol, this induces general feelings of wellbeing throughout your baby's body.
- Promotes attachment. As you massage your baby, you also maintain eye contact, kiss, caress and vocalise, which encourage closeness in a relationship.

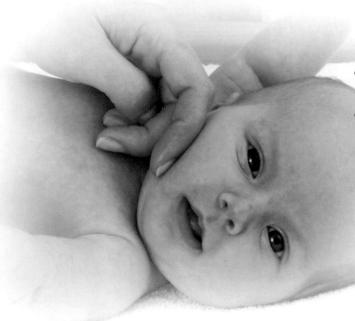

Physical

The skin provides the central nervous system with a continual stream of information about the body's immediate environment. As you touch your baby's skin, the sensation is relayed to her central nervous system, which initiates physical and physiological responses in addition to the emotional ones. Regular massage produces the following physical benefits:

- The healthy growth and development of your baby. Touch is every bit as important as vitamins, minerals and proteins; babies who are deprived of touch do not thrive.
- The increase of growth hormones from the pituitary gland.
- Improved circulation. As muscles relax, they absorb blood and when they contract, they help to pump blood back to the heart and aid the venous return. The periphery of your baby's body—the top of her head and her hands and feet—are often cold because her circulatory system is not fully developed. Massage will warm her hands and feet.

- Muscle relaxation and joint flexibility. Massage enables muscles to relax, and as they do so, they allow the free movement of the body's joints. Joint flexibility is vital in enabling your baby to establish a wide range of physical movements and mobility.
- Cleansing your baby's skin and helping to remove dead cells. Massage opens the pores and encourages the elimination of toxins and the secretion of sebum—the natural oil that aids the skin's elasticity and resilience and resistance to infections.
- Stimulation of the vagus nerve. One branch of this leads to the gastro-intestinal tract, where it facilitates the release of food absorption hormones such as insulin and glucose.
- Promoting the flow of waste-removing lymphatic fluid thus improving the body's resistance to infection.

1 INTRODUCING YOUR BABY TO MASSAGE

From the very beginning, the mother should remain at the center of any "treatment" offered to her baby. Most mothers want to hold their babies and establish skin-to-skin contact before the baby is removed to be weighed, measured, bathed or dressed. From his mother's womb into her arms, touch becomes the primal language of the newborn, and it is through holding and caressing that a baby is made to feel welcomed and loved.

The maternally sensitive period—both physically and emotionally—immediately following a baby's birth is one in which to welcome a new baby quite literally into the bosom of the family. For those mothers and babies who miss this period, however, it also can be created at a later time—and greatly assisted by some of the techniques shown in this book.

The mother and child relationship is like no other. It lays a foundation of love and learning that can affect a child for the rest of his life. By comparison with all other mammals, human babies are premature and they need to be held, rubbed, rocked and talked to for the first eight weeks of life until they have "gathered their senses in a new and unfamiliar environment."

Although the need to be held, stroked and touched continues throughout our lives, it is at its most intense in infancy during the pre-verbal period.

Key benefits of early massage

- Skin-to-skin physical contact stimulates the release of the "love" hormone, oxytocin, and the natural "stress relievers," endorphins and these, in turn, encourage closeness and contentment between parent and baby.

- Developing your sense of touch increases your confidence and makes your baby feel protected and loved. This strengthens the physical and emotional bonds between parent and baby and nurtures your baby's feelings of security.

- Massage assists digestion, relaxes the tummy and encourages feelings of tranquillity.

- Massage strengthens your baby's immune system and will help your baby to breathe deeper, and through continued abdominal breathing, absorb more oxygen for less effort.

Getting in touch

Newborn babies usually spend most of their time sleeping—maybe as many as 18 hours a day—but from about six to eight weeks of age, your baby will still sleep for something like 15 hours a day and (hopefully) more of these hours will be concentrated around night-time. Between feeds, when your baby is not too full and not hungry, but rather has settled into a quiet state of wakefulness, you can start to develop your sense of touch and begin to introduce massage.

As time goes on, your baby's periods of wakefulness will become longer and so your opportunities for massage will be greater. Getting your baby used to being touched and stroked at an early stage will help to make a more formal massage routine far easier and more enjoyable for you both later on.

Most very young babies feel very vulnerable when they are naked, but will respond well to gentle, non-intrusive stroking—first through clothes and at the right time in the right environment, when naked.

When your baby has become used to your touch, has had his six-to-eight week check, and has a fair degree of back and neck strength, you can start to give a more structured massage (see Chapter Two).

Getting in Touch

From the first few days onwards, taking a little time for you and your new baby to literally get the feel of each other will have many benefits. Touch is your baby's "mother sense" and through touch (and smell) your baby will learn quickly to recognize you. Trust and confidence also build in you through handling your baby and in your baby by being handled.

Introducing massage at this time should be as little intrusive as possible and done with your baby clothed.

Try cradling your baby in your arms and gently knead her tummy from side to side with a relaxed cupped hand. Once you get the feel of her tummy, close your eyes and feel the contours of your baby's body. Squeeze very gently her legs and feet, arms, shoulders and chest. Place a relaxed cupped hand across the crown of her head, and then return it to her tummy.

NEWBORN POSTURE
A young baby holds her limbs close to her body with her arms and legs bent. Her head rests to the side as her neck muscles aren't yet strong enough to support it. If your baby holds her limbs tightly into her body you can begin to help her to relax them.

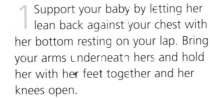

1 Support your baby by letting her lean back against your chest with her bottom resting on your lap. Bring your arms underneath hers and hold her with her feet together and her knees open.

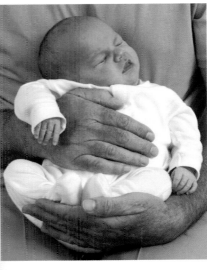

2 Place one hand lightly across her tummy and gently massage her tummy from side to side. Open your other hand to support her lower legs and feet. Leaning back, slowly drop down the hand supporting her legs and feet to encourage your baby to lower her feet and relax and straighten her legs.

NEVER TRY TO FORCE any of the movements. If your baby is not happy with your touches, cradle her in your arms and return to the sequence at another time.

11

3 Now bring your hands over her shoulders and squeeze softly using relaxed open hands.

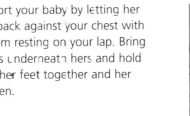

4 With relaxed hands stroke gently down the length of her arms to help relax and straighten them. Then gently lay her facing you with her back resting on your thighs and her legs placed against your tummy, and with her knees open and her feet together, rock her gently.

YOUR BABY MAY FALL ASLEEP as you do this, but if she starts to fuss or cry, always stop and give her a cuddle. Remember, this is something you do with and never to your baby.

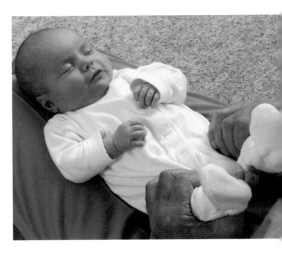

First Stretch

Tranquillity comes from the belly, which is a major emotional center. Keep your baby's tummy relaxed and you will keep your baby relaxed. If your baby's tummy is relaxed, she will breathe more deeply and take in more oxygen for less effort. Belly breathing will provide her with a greater sense of overall relaxation. This is particularly important if your baby has been traumatized or is fractious or anxious, due to trauma during pregnancy, delivery or following birth.

A gentle massage from side to side will help to relax your baby's tummy.

Spending some waking time lying on a relaxed tummy (see pages 18–19) will also relax and prepare your baby for the first stage in her developmental pattern—independently raising her head.

PHYSIOLOGICAL FLEXION

This term describes the tension that pulls your baby into a fetal posture as a result of growing within the confined space of the womb. Once your baby has started to relax, using the positions shown previously, the movements below will help your baby relax more and stretch out more fully from a fetal position (a bit like stretching your own limbs after a good night's sleep).

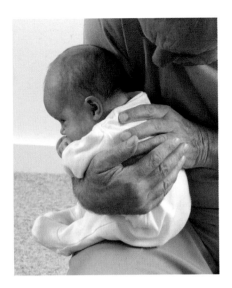

1 Sit in a comfortable chair and place your baby sitting sideways on your lap. Let her lean forwards with her arms extended over your forearm. With relaxed, open hands, gently rub your baby's head and neck stroking down to the base of her spine and up again.

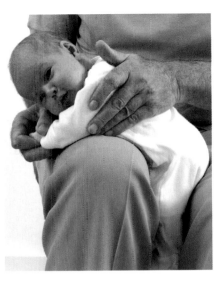

2 Only when your baby has relaxed in position one, gently lay her tummy forward over your thighs. Her arms are extended and her legs supported between yours. Gently rock your baby and gently rub the sides of her upper back and arms (the latissimus dorsi and trapezius muscles) to relax her arms and shoulders.

13

3 Only when your baby is relaxed in position two, rock her gently and straighten her legs over your thighs. Now with your baby fully relaxed and extended in this position, stroke down the length of your baby's back and legs, rubbing and patting and rocking her gently.

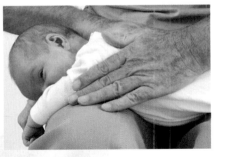

THIS IS A GREAT FIRST HOLDING POSITION which will allow you to hold your baby while leaving your arms and hands free.

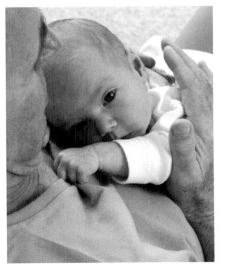

4 Once your baby has fully relaxed, gently slide down on your chair so that your body is inclined. Carefully lift your baby with your hands under her arms and lay her along your chest, in a heart-to-heart position, with her legs extending downwards. Continue to stroke gently down the length of her back.

THE SOUND OF YOUR HEARTBEAT will comfort your baby and now that your baby has stretched her tummy, she will be a more relaxed, calmer and happier baby. Include lots of kisses and *don't forget to show dad*.

Skin-to-Skin Contact

Once your baby is happy to be rubbed, rocked and stroked naked, the skin-to-skin touches will help your baby to feel even more content and further promote the feelings of closeness between the two of you.

Create an environment as welcoming as possible; make the room warm and quiet and lay your baby on a warm, soft, doubled bath towel. Remove your baby's clothes slowly and talk with your baby as you do this. Take off any jewelry that could scratch your baby's skin and make sure your hands are clean and warmed—rub them together and give them a shake to loosen them up before you lay hands on your baby. Keep your movements relaxed and rhythmic.

ESTABLISH EYE CONTACT
Look into your baby's eyes as you begin to caress him and every time he faces you.

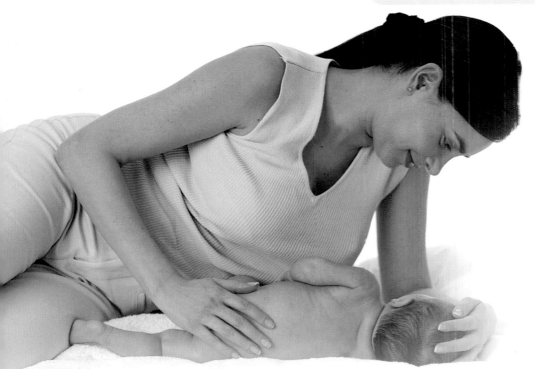

1 Lay down on your left side, with your baby facing you, lying on his right side. Stroke your baby with the whole of your right hand, from the back of his neck to the base of his spine—in the same way as you would stroke a kitten or a puppy.

• **Continue for about a minute.**

2 Use a circular movement to gently massage around your baby's upper back and then right down the length of his back to the base of his spine.

• **Continue for about a minute.**

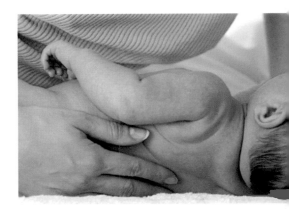

3 Next, slowly take the movement to his arm. Keep your touch gentle and relaxed as you take the stroke from his shoulder to his hand.

• **Continue for about a minute. Repeat with his right arm.**

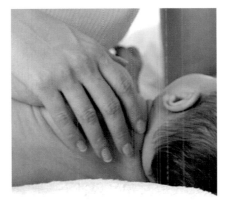

4 Move your hand to the top of your baby's leg and stroke down from his hip to his foot with your palm. You can give his leg a little gentle shake to loosen it up and help him to relax.

• **Continue for about a minute. Repeat with his right leg.**

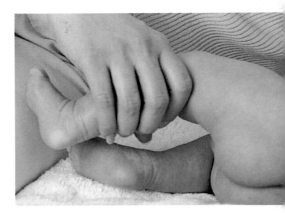

Father and Baby

Fathers don't experience the nine months of physical closeness that mothers share with their babies during that first period of growth and development inside her body. Many mothers feel their babies "fluttering" during the early weeks and as the baby grows larger and turns and presses against the walls of the uterus, movements are felt more and more intensely. From here on, most mothers to be massage their unborn babies through their abdomens to quieten them when they get restless.

The first time a father has direct physical contact with his baby is usually at birth, when the child is handed to him. Touching and holding such a tiny person can be daunting, and it is important for both father and baby to be given ample opportunity to "get in touch."

Fathers benefit from time spent with their babies, and massage can help to develop their touch and handling skills. Practicing the strokes below will foster trust between a father and his child, and increases the father's confidence in his ability to change and bathe his baby and to help more with the daily responsibilities of childcare. Massage will also help to strengthen the physical and emotional relationship between the two. By learning how to handle his baby better, a father is more able to soothe and comfort his baby at times when the baby's mother needs to take a break.

You can adapt the movements shown for any occasion when you are just sitting with your baby. For example, you can stroke your baby's back and around his neck and shoulders as he sits on your lap.

GETTING TO KNOW EACH OTHER
Holding your baby close and whenever possible looking into his eyes will help to build your relationship.

Make sure that you
are laying comfortably
and that your shoulders
are relaxed throughout
the massage.

1 Lay down on your side with your baby facing you,
laying on his side. Using the relaxed weight of your
whole right hand, start stroking your baby's upper
back in a circular motion.

• **TRY AND ESTABLISH EYE CONTACT at the beginning of the
massage and maintain it whenever possible throughout.**

2 Then take this movement down the length of your baby's spine
smoothly, to include your baby's lower back

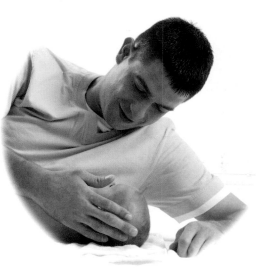

3 Using the palm of your hand, gently stroke
all around the crown of your baby's head in a
slow, circular motion.

• **Repeat for as long as your baby is relaxed and
comfortable.**

17

Introducing Your Baby to Massage

Belly Time

For your young baby, regular waking time spent laying belly-down ensures the structural health and fitness of his body in a way no other natural position can achieve. Ultimately, spending waking time on his belly will make it easier for him to crawl. Babies who do not lay on their bellies usually develop later than those who do.

When your baby lies on his belly, he lifts his head to look around him—strengthening the supporting muscles in his neck. Once he has comfortably reached this stage, he will then lift his head and shoulders, developing strength in his arms and shoulders and flexibility in his spine.

Having achieved this, he will then raise his head and shoulders even further. This stretches open your baby's chest, so that he achieves a deeper breathing rhythm and maximizes his lung capacity. A deeper breathing rhythm is of great benefit to the heart and lungs and the increase of oxygen will also boost all the other major organs and your baby's immune system. And as his chest stretches open, so, too, does his abdominal cavity—aiding digestion.

> To counteract the incidence of sudden infant death syndrome (SIDS), do not lay your baby on his belly to sleep. However, periods spent laying on his belly during waking time will promote your baby's development.

To complete this gradual phase of development, your baby will lift his head, chest, arms and shoulders and, ultimately, his legs and feet in a unique display of strength and flexibility. It is important to encourage your baby to spend some waking time lying on his belly, so if your baby initially finds it uncomfortable, use the technique set out below.

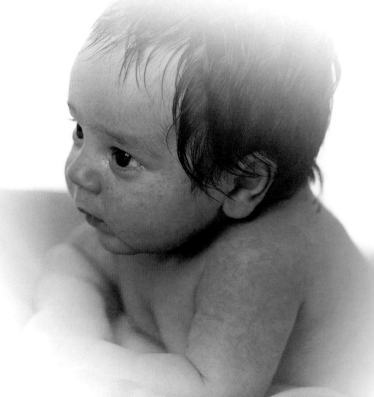

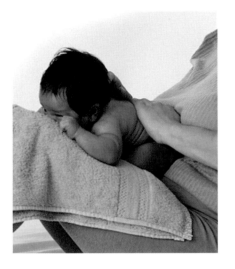

1 Sit comfortably against a wall with your knees bent. Lay your baby belly down on your thighs, with his knees open and his feet together. Make sure that his feet are pressed together.

CHECK THAT YOUR BABY'S FEET ARE NOT FLAT AGAINST YOUR BELLY; in this position he can push against you and propel himself over your knees.

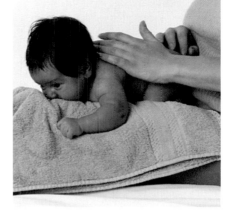

2 Stroke your baby's back, hand-over-hand, and make him feel comfortable in this position, then very gradually lower your knees.

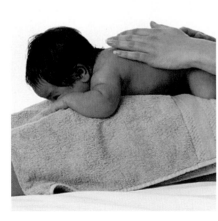

3 Keep bringing your knees down very slowly until your baby is eventually laying flat on your thighs. Keep stroking his back throughout.

4 When your baby is comfortable with this, you can lay him belly down on a towel on the floor. Support his chest and shoulders on a cushion. Soon you will be able to remove the cushion, giving your baby the full benefits of time on his belly.

AIR BATHING

Babies need to spend time naked so that their skin is exposed to fresh air. Known as "air bathing" this is beneficial for maintaining the skin's health and resilience to infection. Once you regularly massage your baby, you will ensure that her skin is consistently air bathed, but even when you are not massaging, you can allow her to spend time naked around the house and, more importantly, outside. By doing this, you are allowing your baby's skin to absorb the life-sustaining and healing properties of oxygen and absorb natural light—major components in the skin's production of vitamin D, which calcifies newly formed bone protein to create stronger bones.

Those times when your baby really isn't ready for or doesn't fancy a massage aren't lost if your baby is still given the opportunity to enjoy a greater freedom of movement, unhampered by the restrictions of clothes.

Of course, you must make sure that the temperature is comfortable for your naked baby and that she is protected from the sun. If your baby is naked outside, ensure that it is sufficiently warm, with no cool breezes, but that she is out of direct or reflected sunlight. If you are inside, choose a warm, well-ventilated room and keep her away from any draughts. Take care to supervise her at all times.

LIGHT THERAPY
From two months, most babies love being naked. Bathing the skin in oxygen and light can help to prevent and cure any minor skin disorders such as nappy rash.

1 Encourage your baby to hold
her feet and suck her toes—
look at the wonderful range of
movement she has.

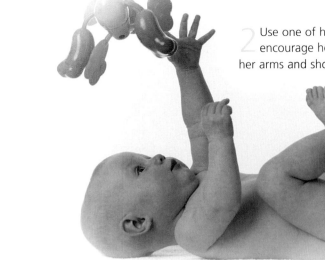

2 Use one of her favorite toys to
encourage her to stretch out
her arms and shoulders.

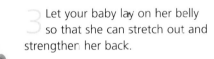

3 Let your baby lay on her belly
so that she can stretch out and
strengthen her back.

4 Once she is comfortable, she
will strengthen herself even
more by pulling her arms and
shoulders back.

Introducing Your Baby to Massage

2 TOE-TO-TOP MASSAGE

From about two months of age, your baby should be feeling a little less vulnerable. It is likely that he will feel happy to remain naked and has lost some of the physiological flexion that kept his arms and legs tucked into his body in a semi-fetal posture as a newborn. When he has reached this stage, you can start to introduce the following complete body massage routine, which will help him to achieve his maximum potential at each phase of development during the following months.

Most babies prefer massage to begin with their feet and legs and continue up the body, as this is a non-invasive and gradual approach, which allows your baby to get used to the routine. Starting at your baby's feet and continuing fluidly up his body, this comprehensive sequence of massage techniques can secure your baby's full structural health and fitness. It encourages the flexibility of all of his major joints, relaxes his muscles and will provide him with a solid foundation for good posture and later mobility.

The routine should be practiced regularly—every day if possible—giving you and your baby a regular period of special time and closeness.

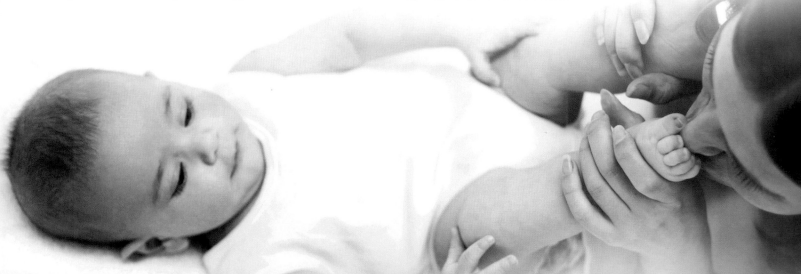

Key benefits of full-body massage

- Maintains balance and posture through the right order of strength and flexibility.

- Improves muscular coordination and suppleness and relieves muscle and joint inflexibility.

- Releases any hidden areas of tension in muscles and re-aligns the joints.

- Promotes the flexibility of the spine and strength in the muscles that support it.

- Aids digestion and tranquillity by allowing the belly to relax more easily.

- Maximizes breathing volume to promote wellbeing; more oxygen and good circulation will help your baby to thrive.

- Promotes the integrity and alignment of all the major joints and good tone in the muscle groups that control them.

- Cleanses the skin and exposes it to light and oxygen.

Choose the time of day when your baby is at his best—not too full, too hungry or too tired. Above all else, this is something you do with your baby, not to your baby, so take your cues from him and punctuate your massage with lots of hugs and kisses.

You do not have to perform the sequence all in one go—introduce it a little at a time—but aim to graduate to a full session. The separate massage techniques are designed to interlink, so that all the major muscles and joints are included.

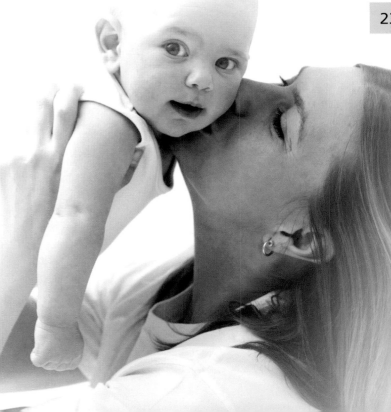

TOUCHES AND TECHNIQUES

When you massage your baby, you need to keep your hands open and relaxed and make contact with your baby's skin with your fingers and your palms. If your hands are stiff and your touch is hesitant, you may transfer tension to your baby, so try to remain relaxed and confident by breathing with your belly and relaxing your hands arms and shoulders.

As your baby develops and enjoys a more formal massage routine, you can increase the pressure slightly to give a little more depth to your touch. This gives your baby an important message—he is resilient. The more confident your touch, the more confidence you instill in your baby. And as your baby develops, you may need to increase the speed of your strokes to hold his attention and keep him engaged.

Punctuate your massage with lots of hugs and kisses, talk and sing to your baby and enjoy it. Babies love to play—this is how they learn best. As soon as you start to get too serious, your baby will lose interest in the massage and disengage.

Keep your hands on your baby's skin as much as you can and, if you stop to turn a page in this book, or to replenish your oil, keep one hand resting upon your baby's body.

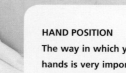

HAND POSITION
The way in which you use your hands is very important and will make all the difference to the effectiveness of your baby's massage.

The strokes themselves are not difficult to learn and you will soon be doing them intuitively. Rub your hands together and give them a shake to warm them and loosen them up before you start. Keep your hands relaxed from your wrists. The main terms to look out for are as follows:

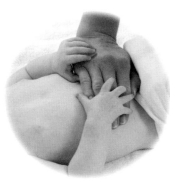

Knead
Squeeze and release the soft parts of your baby's body gently with your whole hand.

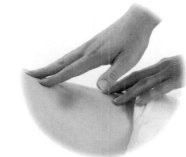

Stroke
Move the relaxed weight of your whole hand across the surface of your baby's body.

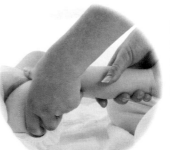

Hand-over-hand
Begin a movement with one hand as you cease the same movement with the other hand.

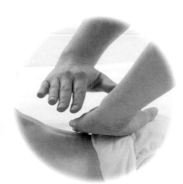

Percussion
Use the relaxed weight of your cupped hands to tap rhythmically on the front or back of the body.

Rub
Press gently and move the relaxed weight of your hand or hands backwards and forwards over your baby's body or limb.

Massage Oils

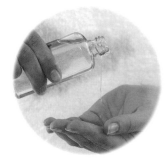

Your baby's skin is fine and sensitive, with far more nerve endings than that of any adult. The constant regeneration of healthy cells keeps your baby's skin smooth and moist and a regular massage with an appropriate oil will also cleanse the skin's pores of its dead cells and give it a healthy glow. The oil that you use should allow your hands to glide easily and enable you to give more depth to your touch without discomfort. It should not be highly perfumed nor should it feel too sticky or greasy. It should be pure in its content and whenever possible, organic.

Base oils

Base or carrier oils are unperfumed and derived from nuts, seeds and pulp, etc. They often have therapeutic properties on their own—olive oil, for example, is a good moisturiser—but they also can be used to dilute essential oils. Natural fruit or vegetable oils are readily absorbed through the surface of the skin, so you will need to keep replenishing your supply as you massage. The following oils are inexpensive and widely available:

- *Grapeseed* A fine oil, it is known for its purity and easy absorption.
- *Olive oil* Rich and good for dry skin.
- *Sunflower oil* (organic only) A fine, odorless oil, it is highly recommended and can be used with premature babies.

Do not use Aracas oil as it is derived from peanuts and your baby may be allergic. Sweet almond is also a nut oil, so it is no longer recommended.

Essential oils

These are highly refined oils that possess the scent and the healing properties of the plant, flower or herb from which they were extracted. They contain natural chemical constituents, which can be used to help promote and maintain health and wellbeing. Each essential oil has unique therapeutic properties. The oils are highly potent, however, and are not recommended for use with very young babies. Before eight weeks of age, they should not be used at all on your baby (although you can use a recommended base oil). Once your baby is eight weeks old, oils can be effective, but they should only be used if they are well diluted—two drops of essential oil to three tablespoons of base massage oil. Because your baby is "aroma sensitive," check first that he has no adverse reaction to the blend. Many unexplained episodes of crying are related to highly perfumed oils in aftershaves, cosmetics, household air fresheners and furniture polish. Your baby's sense of smell is what binds him to you. As such it is acutely sensitive.

Not all essential oils are suitable for babies but some of the most useful and effective are:

- *Ravensara* Non-toxic and antiseptic, this is good for viral and skin infections and nappy rash.

- *Chamomile Roman* Calming and soothing, this oil aids digestion and soothes irritability (see page 84). May be helpful for treating colic.
- *Lavender* This antiseptic oil is good for soothing and healing minor burns and bites. It can also be used as a chest or nasal decongestant (see page 78).
- *Eucalyptus* A powerful decongestant, it can be used for a chest-and-back massage (see page 78) to relieve coughs, colds and congestion. Do not use if your baby is having homoeopathic treatment.

Always "skin test" the oil you intend to use. Rub a little into a small area of skin on the top of your baby's arm, and wait for one hour to see if there is any allergic reaction. This may look like a heat rash or red blotches, which will disappear after an hour or two. Should this happen, try another oil.

- *Frankincense* Deeply relaxing with a very pleasant aroma, it can also be used for a chest massage (see page 38) to deepen the breathing rhythm and soothe discomfort. Can promote sleep.
- *Rose otto* Recommended for dry skin, it has a beautiful aroma but is expensive.

Herbal oils

These are oils created by infusing fresh or dried herbs in a vegetable oil. Ones beneficial to mother and baby are:

- *Arnica* Can help to heal bruising.
- *Lime blossom* Encourages sleep.
- *Calendula* A very healing and soothing oil, it is particularly gentle on skin and can help soothe nappy rash and moisturise dry skin.

Using oils

Pour the oil into a saucer so that it is not easily spilled. Make sure that the saucer is within reaching distance, so that you can replenish your oil easily as you massage.

When ready to massage, dip your fingers in the oil and rub your hands together to spread the oil between your palms. Rubbing the palms also warms the oil. Reapply when your hands feel dry or they stop gliding smoothly over your baby's skin.

Never pour the remaining oil back into the bottle, as it may now be contaminated.

Buying and storing oils

Choose pure and natural oils, preferably organic, and from a reputable supplier. Essential oils should be packaged in dark coloured glass, since this filters out the sun's ultra-violet light.

Choose a cool, dark and dry place to keep oils safely away from heat and inquisitive children. Never leave oils where the sun will shine directly on them—like on a window shelf—because they will deteriorate rapidly.

Particularly in summer, carrier and massage oils can benefit by being refrigerated. You will need to allow them to warm up before use; let stand for a few hours to return to room temperature. Some carrier oils form fatty particles at low temperatures, which will need to be dissolved again before you can use them. A quick shake of the bottle is all that is needed to return them to their normal condition.

Before You Begin

Treat your massage sessions as special times and create a pleasant environment for the massage. Use a quiet, warm, draught-free room in which you can remain uninterrupted for about an hour. If your room is not carpeted, lay a soft towel over a sheepskin or a folded blanket for your baby. Your baby will not feel comfortable on a hard surface and, if he lacks head control, he could bump his head. If your room is carpeted, use a soft, thick cotton towel for your baby. Avoid wool as it can irritate your baby's skin. You will need a cushion to sit on and perhaps you and your baby may also find some soft music relaxing.

KNEEL DOWN AND SIT COMFORTABLY ON YOUR FEET on a cushion with your knees open. Relax your arms and shoulders.

Have your saucer of massage oil within easy reach and a nappy and a fresh towel handy as your baby may pee during the massage. Your baby may well wish to feed after his massage, so if you are bottle-feeding, have a prepared bottle close to hand.

Relax, enjoy and have fun; massage is meant to be pleasurable for you both. Try to stay calm calm and focused; breathing with your belly may help with this. Try not to get distracted or hurried, as this may prevent your baby responding well. If this does happen and your baby gets upset, always stop and give him a feed or a cuddle and then, if you feel inclined, try again—perhaps with him clothed. Babies who resist massage are often ones who need it the most and end up most enjoying it.

- Wear comfortable, loose-fitting clothes.
- Wash your hands and make sure that they are not cold; remove any jewelry that could scratch your baby's skin.
- Apply oil as and when necessary.
- Keep your touch rhythmic and put your mind in your hands. Put aside worries and focus on what you are doing as you do it.
- Talk and sing to your baby and try to maintain eye contact.
- Always stop if your baby cries. This is something that you do with your baby, not to your baby.

When to massage

Choosing the right time to massage your baby can make all the difference as to whether or not he will enjoy it. A good time to massage is last thing at night, after your baby's bath, or any time during the day when he is at his most relaxed and responsive. Don't massage him just after a feed; if he is too full, the process can be uncomfortable, especially when you are massaging his belly or laying him on his front to massage his back. Don't massage him either when he is hungry; he is unlikely to tolerate being massaged for any length of time if he wants to be fed.

Try to be consistent with the timing of your massage, so that your baby will learn to anticipate and look forward to the sessions.

If your baby does not immediately seem to respond well, persevere—three or four sessions is usually all it takes for babies to begin enjoying massage. You do not need to Practice the whole of a sequence straight away; stop when your baby wants to and build your routine little by little each session.

Postures

It is important that you remain relaxed and that your position is comfortable while you are massaging your baby. The sitting positions shown can be fairly easily maintained, but however you sit, make sure that you can lean forward without straining your back. If you do become uncomfortable at any point during a massage, pause the massage and change your position.

When not to massage

- With the exception of the massages specifically designed to alleviate the symptoms of discomfort (see Chapter Five), do not massage your baby if he is unwell. In most cases, babies who are feeling ill just want to sleep and be held but may respond well to having their feet and/or hands rubbed.
- You should never massage your baby against his will and best not to wake him for a massage.
- Do not massage your baby with oil if he has a weeping skin condition, as the oil may exacerbate it. Consult your physician for advice and a suitable alternative.
- If your baby has been immunised, wait for 48 hours to find out how he has been affected. Avoid the site of the injection, but if it leaves a hard lump, you can gently knead it away between your thumb and forefinger once it is no longer sensitive.
- Avoid any areas of your baby's body that are bruised, swollen, at all inflamed or acutely sensitive. Consult your physician before massaging.

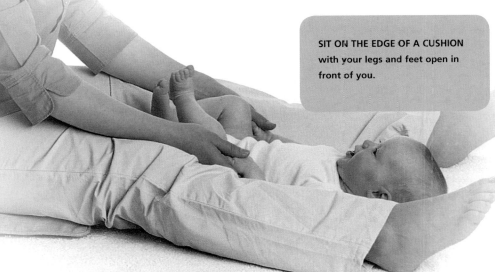

SIT ON THE EDGE OF A CUSHION with your legs and feet open in front of you.

29

Toe-to-Top Massage

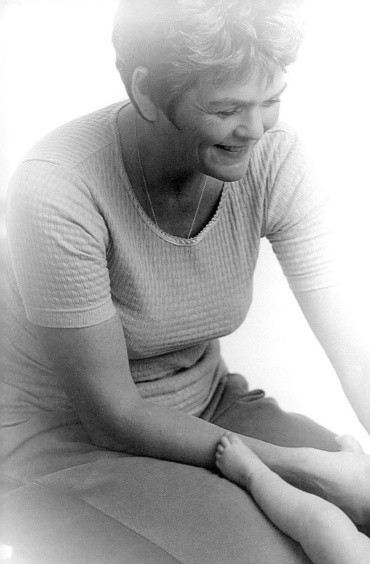

Feet...

Foot massage is one of the oldest forms of massage and can be extremely relaxing for the whole body. Your baby will find it pleasurable and it will also help with her balance and posture as she spreads her toes, extends her heels and opens her feet.

The soles of your baby's feet are very sensitive and stroking them will provoke a reflex—she will curl her toes. As a result, you should concentrate on the less ticklish tops and sides of the feet. Stroking the top of her toes and the outer side of her ankles will encourage your baby to extend her toes, so focus on these areas for the best effect.

When your baby gets a little older and starts walking, you should allow her to enjoy the freedom of being barefooted for the first six weeks before putting her in shoes, so that her feet can develop, spread and assume their natural shape. To stand with confidence and security, your baby's heels must be well-grounded. This is why it is best not to encourage your baby to stand on tiptoes—the more she stands on her toes, the more insecure she will feel and the more difficult she will find it to balance. The following technique will help your baby to open her feet and bring down her heels in preparation for standing—this is particularly important if her feet tend to turn inwards.

EASY ACCESS
You can massage your baby's feet anywhere you happen to be together and even when she is wearing socks. (Gently massaging your baby's feet while clothed can be non-obtrusive and very soothing if she is unwell.)

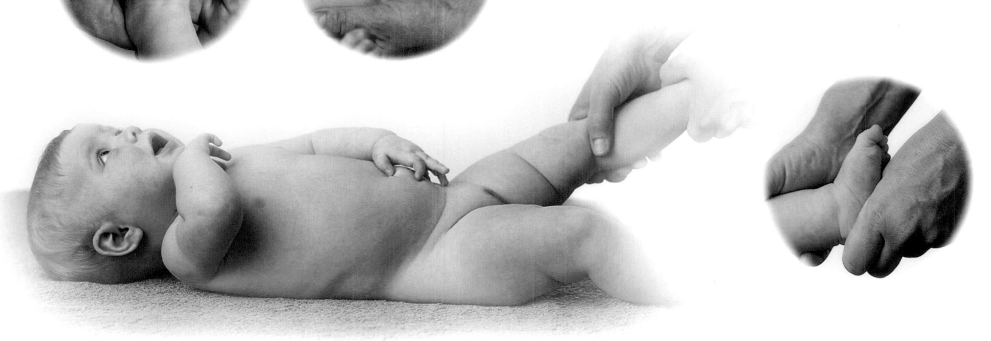

1 Make sure that your hands are well oiled. Begin to knead and rub the top of your baby's foot with your hands.

• **Continue for 2–3 minutes.**

2 Then, start to roll each toe between your forefinger and thumb and gently separate the toes so that they fan out slightly.

• **Continue for about 20 seconds.**

Toe-to-Top Massage

3 Now pull the whole foot smoothly, hand-over-hand, through your palms. You will probably need to replenish your oil at this stage of the massage.

• **Continue for about 20 seconds.**

4 Flex your baby's ankle and extend the heel of her foot by turning her foot outwards with one hand while you rub her calf with the other.

• **Continue for about 20 seconds. Repeat with the other foot.**

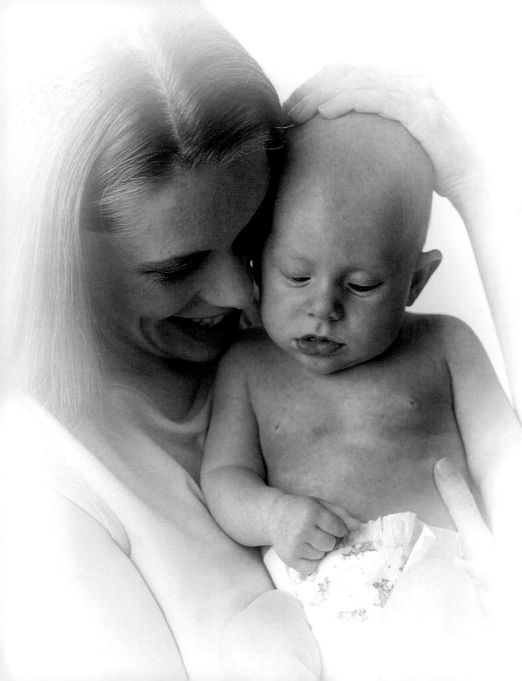

...to Legs...

From about two months, your baby will begin to exercise his legs vigorously, kicking and stretching them daily for hours on end in a wonderful display of aerobics. This develops the strength and coordination of his postural muscles—the calves, thighs and buttocks—and secures and maintains the flexibility of his hips and knees. The strength and coordination of these muscles and the flexibility of these joints will provide your baby with a strong foundation for upright postures and a wide variety of movement.

Both sitting and standing involve balance and this is made far easier when flexible joints provide your baby with a broad base. Your baby will develop the self-confidence to stand tall with the inner feeling that the foundations of his body—his legs—are both strong and flexible.

Massaging your baby's legs will help to promote the development of coordination, strengthen his lower back and maintain the flexibility of his knees and ankles. It will also ensure that there are no areas of hidden tension or stiffness in any of his muscles and joints.

INCREASED FLEXIBILITY
These massage techniques will leave your baby's legs completely relaxed and supple.

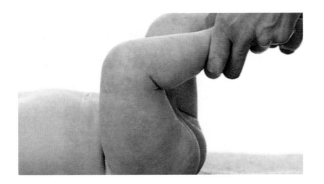 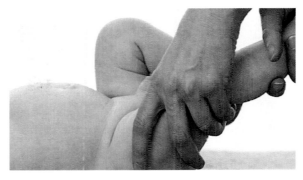 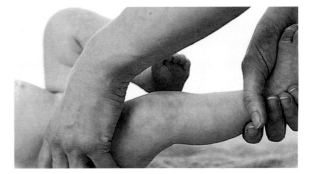

1 Hold both of your baby's legs by the ankles and loosen them up a little by gently "bicycling" them, bending and straightening them alternately.
• **Continue for about 20 seconds.**

2 Then put your left hand at the top of your baby's right leg and pull through your well-oiled palms from his thigh downwards in a hand-over-hand movement, right down to his foot.
• **Repeat 4–5 times.**

3 Hold your baby's right ankle in your right hand and massage his thigh with your left hand. Massage up the front, then down the back of his thigh.
• **Repeat 4–5 times.**

4 Now, pull the whole leg again from the thigh to the foot hand-over-hand.
• **Repeat the sequence with your baby's left leg.**

5 Shake your baby's legs and rest your hands on his inner thighs. Turn your hands outwards and pull down the back of his knees and calves—he will straighten his legs. Keep gliding your hands up the front and down the back of his legs.
• **Repeat 4–5 times.**

...to Hips...

The flexibility of your baby's hips is crucial for good posture because her upper body bends forward from these joints and they also support her spine and pelvis. Hip mobility is vital to maintaining the integrity of your baby's spine.

Babies enjoy an incredible range of hip movement—they can they hold their feet and suck their toes effortlessly. Some babies, however, can lack this range of movement and for various reasons, others can lose it very early. Massaging your baby's hips in the way shown in this book, will help her to maintain the flexibility of these joints and, once on her feet, to strengthen flexible hip joints. Consistent practice of developmental baby massage will ensure that your baby continues to enjoy a wide variety of movement and maintains good posture, both sitting and standing, as she strengthens.

Although your baby's hips will have been examined at birth, you can make sure that they are developing healthily by checking that they do not "clunk" when she moves, that she can freely open her knees sideways, that both knees look the same when held together and bent and that the two little creases at the bottom of her spine are uniform when she lays down on her belly.

PREVENTING HIP INFLEXIBILITY
Babies who practice standing before they are sitting properly are more prone to hip inflexibility. If your baby likes to stand, complement this with the following massage two or three times a week.

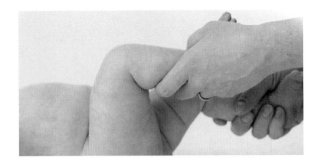

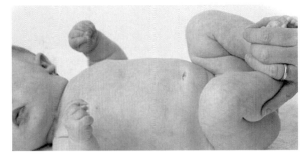

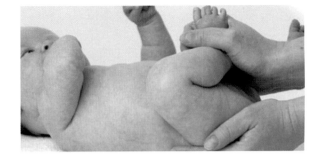

1 Lay your baby on her back and hold her legs by the ankles. Make sure that her legs are relaxed by "bicycling" them a few times—gently bending and straightening them rhythmically one after the other.

• **Continue for about 20 seconds.**

2 Now, clap your baby's feet together and let her knees bend outwards.

• **Continue for about 20 seconds.**

3 Using your right hand, let her knee bend outwards and take your baby's right foot onto her tummy. Hold the foot down gently onto her navel. Keep your right hand in this position while you knead and rub her right buttock and the back of her thigh with your left hand. Do this for about half a minute and then slowly and gently shake your baby's leg straight.

• **Repeat the sequence with your baby's left leg.**

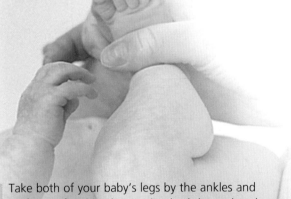

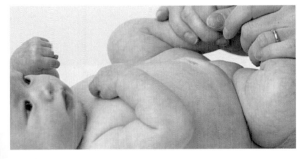

4 Take both of your baby's legs by the ankles and perform a few bicycles. Letting both knees bend outwards clap the soles of her feet together. Push both of your baby's feet down onto her belly. Gently hold her feet in place with your left hand, place your right hand on her lower back and massage around the base of her spine.

• **Continue for about 20 seconds.**

5 Gently shake her legs—bending them and straightening them—and finish by stroking down the front of your baby's legs from the hips to the feet, using the weight of your relaxed hands.

• **Repeat 4–5 times.**

Be sure to perform the steps in the order they are given. Never force any of the movements and if your baby finds any of the positions uncomfortable, consult your doctor.

...to Belly...

Every emotional feeling is mirrored by a change in our muscles and nowhere is this more apparent than in the belly—the emotional center of the body. All our emotions are felt in our bellies and the tummy tightens in response to fear, anxiety and other extreme emotions. Lay your hand on your baby's tummy when she is relaxed and happy and it will feel soft and malleable; do the same when she is upset, and it will be hard and unyielding.

The belly is also a center of tranquillity and massaging your baby's belly in the way shown in this book, will help her to relax and become calmer. It can also relieve stress, infant anxiety and birth trauma. A relaxed belly eases digestion, as it allows the diaphragm at the base of the lungs to descend, both increasing the volume of oxygen and creating a gentle internal wave that soothes the digestive organs with every breath. Managing your baby's tummy in this way can also help to relieve colic and constipation.

Do not try to massage your baby's tummy if she is upset; try instead Tiger in the Tree (see page 88)—a very special technique for crying babies.

TICKLE TREATMENT
If your baby still resists having her belly massaged, pat it, tickle it and loosen it up first, then just lay your hand on it briefly. Once your baby accepts this, you can progress to a full massage.

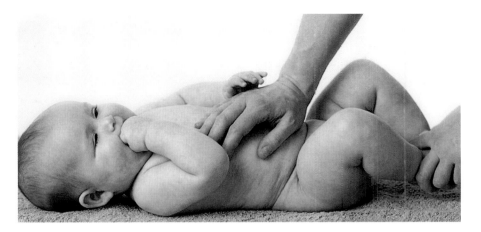

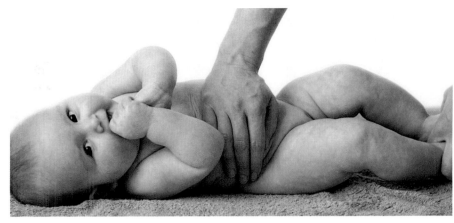

1 Using just the weight of your relaxed hand, massage from your left to your right, in a circular motion. Don't "stroke" the skin but move your hand and your baby's tummy together, kneading the tummy gently and harmoniously clockwise.

• **Repeat 4–5 times.**

2 Place your cupped hand horizontally across your baby's belly and using a relaxed cupped hand, gently knead your baby's tummy from side to side between the lower ribs and the hips. Never push downwards or squeeze the belly hard, as this can cause extreme discomfort.

• **Continue for about 20 seconds.**

3 Massage hand-over-hand, from between the hip and lower ribs on the left side of your baby's body, downwards and across to just below the navel.

• **Repeat several times on each side.**

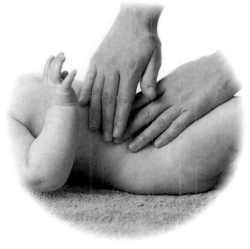

4 As your baby relaxes her tummy, she can release trapped wind and she may urinate. If her stools are loose, she may defecate. So keep a nappy handy and do not over react as this will cause your baby to get upset.

• **Continue for about 20 seconds.**

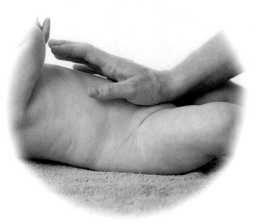

...to Chest...

Oxygen is the very spirit of life and the deeper we breathe, the better we feel. As adults, when we receive an emotional or physical shock, we spontaneously take a deep breath or "gasp," and when we are in a state of stress (marked by a shallow, rapid breathing rhythm), we take controlled breaths in order to calm down. This helps us to maintain a feeling of relaxation and wellbeing as the cells of our bodies receive a plentiful supply of revitalising oxygen.

Your baby's abdominal breathing rhythm is intuitively healthy—her lower ribs and belly expand on the in-breath as she fills her lungs with air and they contract in harmony as she empties them. Your young baby will start to breathe more deeply as she stretches open her chest, arms and shoulders and begins to strengthen and straighten her back in preparation for upright postures and mobility. You can encourage her to maintain her healthy breathing rhythm and reap the benefits of abdominal breathing. An open chest and a relaxed breathing rhythm not only will sustain your baby's growth and development but will help her to resist and recover from illness and infection. Developmental baby massage will encourage your baby to maintain her healthy breathing rhythm and enjoy the benefits of abdominal breathing.

In addition, muscular tension in the chest and tummy can result from repressed or prolonged crying. By mobilizing your baby's chest and rib cage through massage, you enable her to breathe more deeply and efficiently, to gain more oxygen with less effort.

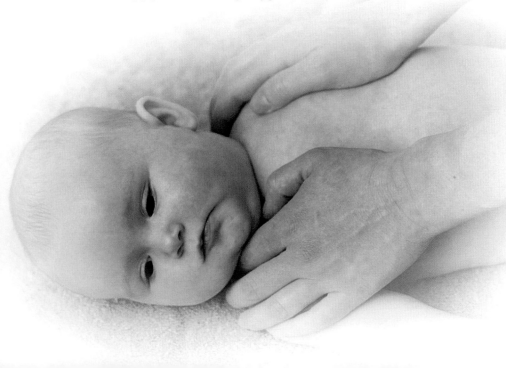

IMPROVED BREATHNG
A regular chest massage will help to open your baby's chest and shoulders.

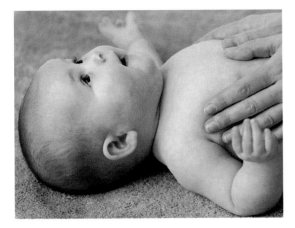

1 Sitting comfortably, with your baby lying on the floor in front of you, place your relaxed well-oiled hands on the center of your baby's chest.

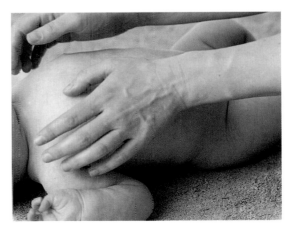

2 Now, with relaxed open hands, massage downwards and outwards around the lower rib cage and return your hands to the center.
• **Repeat 4–5 times.**

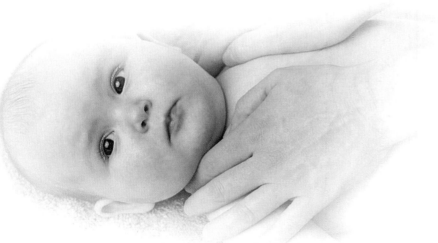

3 Place your hands on the center of your baby's chest and massage upwards and outwards over her shoulders and return you hands to the center again.
• **Repeat 4–5 times.**

4 Cup your hands and tap them lightly across the top and around the sides of your baby's chest in a percussion movement.
• **Continue for about 20 seconds.**

39

Toe-to-Top Massage

...to Shoulders and Arms...

A newborn baby keeps her arms folded and tucked into her chest or the sides of her body. She does not open them readily and it may be some time before she is willing or able to do so. In response to a sudden sound she will throw open her arms involuntarily and draw them back together as if in an embrace. This is the "startle reflex," which will gradually disappear between two and three months as controlled movement takes over.

Voluntarily opening the arms involves a degree of strength and coordination and usually takes two or three months to acquire. During the normal course of development, your baby starts to open her arms downwards, then outwards and then upwards. The outwards movement opens and relaxes the shoulders and chest, while simultaneously closing and strengthening the upper back from side to side. Stretching upwards—lifting the arms and hands above the head—opens the chest and closes and strengthens the upper back downwards, from top to bottom.

Massaging your baby's shoulders and arms in the order of her natural development will ensure full flexibility of her shoulders and suppleness in the muscles of her arms.

LOOSENING UP BABY'S HANDS
Don't forget to play while you massage—hold your baby's hands and give her arms a little shake to loosen them up slightly and kiss and blow on your baby's chest.

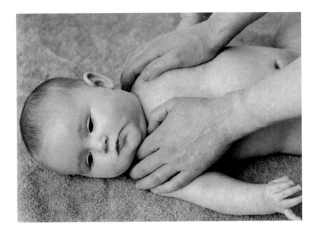

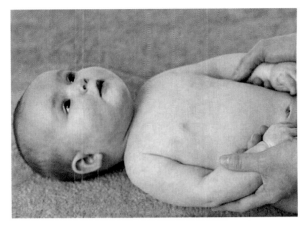

You can encourage your baby to open her arms outwards by clapping her hands together very quickly, which will relax her, before you open her arms.

1 Lay your baby on her back in front of you and, with well-oiled hands, work from the top of your baby's chest, moving your hands upwards and outwards over her shoulders and back to the center.
• **Continue for about 20 seconds.**

2 Move your hands up and outwards over your baby's shoulders and gently pull her arms downwards—in line with her body—through the center of your palms. Keeping in contact, glide your hands back to the top of her chest.
• **Repeat 4–5 times.**

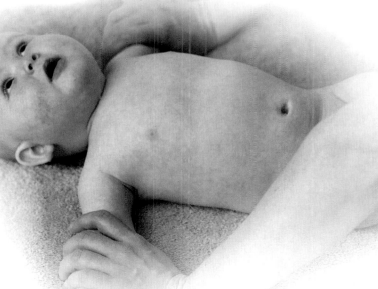

3 Working from the top of her chest, move your hands outwards over your baby's shoulders and gently and smoothly pull her arms outwards in line with her shoulders. Glide your hands back to the top of her chest.
• **Repeat 4–5 times and kiss and blow on your baby's chest.**

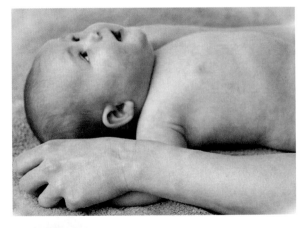

4 Only when your baby is completely comfortable with the first three steps can you take the movement further. Place your hands around the sides of your baby's chest, under her arms, and gently pull her arms upwards through your palms, so that they are above your baby's head. Keep your hands on your baby's skin and glide them lightly back to her chest.
• **Repeat 4–5 times.**

...to Hands...

As instruments of touch, our hands are the most wonderful organs of perception. When we speak of our sense of touch, we associate it almost exclusively with our hands. So much of the quality of our everyday lives depends upon the skillful use of our hands as we use them in a variety of ways—for holding, creating, caressing and communicating.

A young baby lacks the strength and coordination to use her hands efficiently. However, if you put your finger into a newborn's hand, her fingers will close tightly around it—an involuntary movement known as the "grasp reflex." This will disappear between two and three months of age as your baby's hands become more relaxed and open and able to hold onto objects placed in them.

It will be some time before your baby is able to judge distances accurately enough to reach out to grab toys and hold onto them—this usually begins to happen at about five months. And at around six months, your baby may be able to hold her bottle as she drinks, then begin to transfer objects from one hand to the other and, by seven months, she may be able to hold and eat a biscuit by herself. It will be another two months or so before your baby is able to pick up small objects between her thumb and her forefinger and yet another two to three months before she can put an object in your hand and release it.

Massaging your baby's hands is not only fun but can inspire coordination and help your baby to relax her hands and open her fingers.

> **REACHING AND GRASPING**
> The desire to hold objects—manifested when your baby stares intently at her hands—is apparent long before she has the skill to reach out and grasp them.

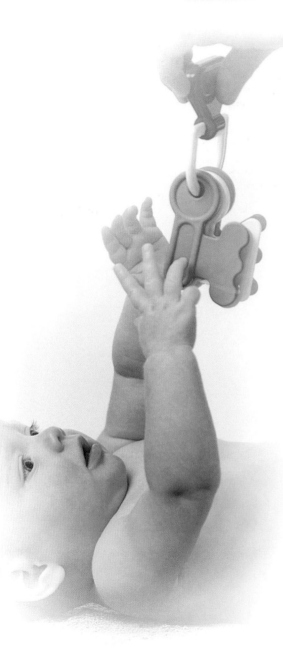

1 Start by opening your baby's hand and rubbing it between your palms.

• **Continue for about 20 seconds.**

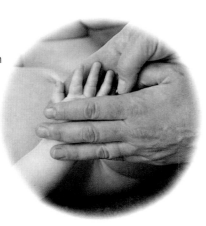

2 Now, relax her hand further by massaging her palm and the back of her hand with your thumbs and index fingers. Work from the wrist to the fingers, squeezing gently backwards and forwards.

• **Repeat 3–4 times.**

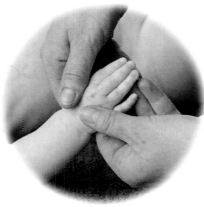

If you use oil for this massage, make sure it is digestible, organic and non-aromatic, like sunflower or grapeseed, and wipe your baby's hands when you have finished; babies are always sucking on their fingers.

43

3 Spread your baby's fingers and thumb and, one by one, gently pull each of them through your thumb and forefinger.

• **Continue for about 20 seconds.**

4 Now rub her whole hand again—back and front—through your palms.

• **Repeat the whole sequence with her other hand.**

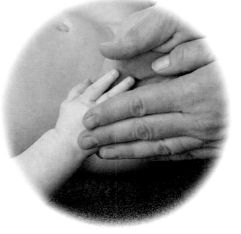

...to Back and Spine...

The spine is of paramount importance in the body's skeletal framework—the head is supported by it, the vital organs are suspended from it and the limbs are attached to it. The spine also houses the body's central nervous system and is the source of all movement. The integrity of your baby's spine thus plays a major role in her health and fitness, both as a child and later as an adult.

Your baby starts to prepare her body for upright postures in the first weeks of her life, but her back muscles really begin to strengthen when she lays on her tummy and starts to lift her head. At this stage, your baby starts to "ground" herself on her tummy and, step-by-step, she will lift her head, chest, shoulders, arms and legs from the floor, eventually attaining a vital developmental posture known as "swimming."

Massaging your baby through the natural phase of swimming will ensure that her back and spine are both strong and flexible, and that she develops excellent posture and a well-balanced body. It will also stretch the front of her body, to maintain a relaxed tummy and her natural abdominal breathing rhythm.

GETTING CLOSE
Kiss your baby's head and blow on her shoulders and spine from time to time—make the massage fun for both of you!

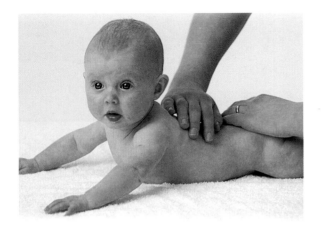

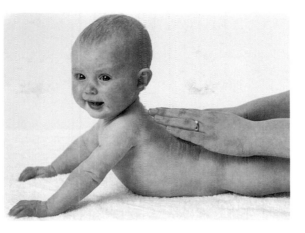

Only do this once your baby can lift her head, chest and shoulders up from the floor in a tummy-forward position with both arms straight. Do not try to lift your baby up; instead, take her hands to her hips. Your baby must lift up herself—when she is ready.

1 Rub plenty of oil into your hands. As your baby lies on her tummy, massage hand-over-hand down her back—from her shoulders down the length of her spine. Use long, firm strokes, but keep your hands relaxed and make it fun for your baby, maybe giving her a tickle now and again!

• **Repeat 4–5 times.**

2 Cup your hands slightly, and pat your baby quite firmly all over her back and shoulders, and up and down the entire length of her spine. Everyone loves a pat on the back and your baby is no exception!

• **Continue for about 20 seconds.**

4 Place both of your hands on the front of your baby's chest and gently pull her shoulders back to open her chest. Follow this movement through to pull her arms back, in line with her body, through the center of your palms, and release gently. Your baby will remain in this position on her own accord before bringing her arms forward again..

• **Repeat 3–4 times.**

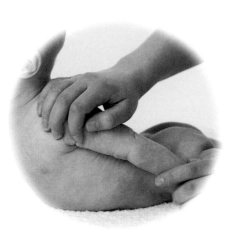

3 When your baby can rest her weight on straight arms, you can develop the massage. Put one well-oiled hand on the center of your baby's chest, and draw it back across the front of her left shoulder and down her arm a couple of times. Make sure to keep her arm alongside her chest and to take her hand to her hip and not to lift it up.

• **Repeat with her right arm.**

...to Head and Neck

The crown of your baby's head fits perfectly into the palm of your hand and because you need to support the head when you hold your baby, it is the most obvious part of the body to massage. Head and neck massage is calming and extremely relaxing, and can be done almost anywhere and any time. It is remarkably effective—instantly soothing—and completely non-intrusive. No prior preparation is needed: your baby does not have to be undressed and you do not need to use any massage oil.

Your baby's head has a number of fibrous joints called suturas which, due to their ability to move slightly, enabled his head to pass through the birth canal. The fontanelle or soft spot left behind on the top of his head is a strong membrane, but massage it gently, stroking with your fingertips and the palm of your hand. Some babies' heads are marked or bruised during delivery—wait for any obvious injury to subside before you begin to massage.

SEATED MASSAGE
Sit in a comfortable chair with your baby on your lap. An armrest will make it possible for you to rest your arm, if needed.

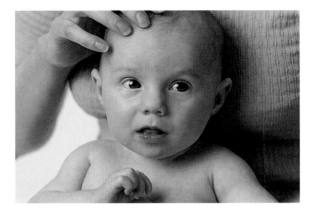

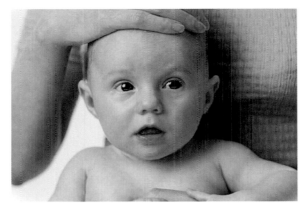

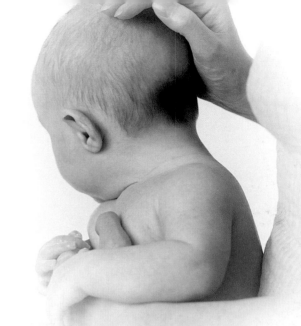

1 Start by lightly massaging around the top of your baby's head in a circular direction with the tips of your fingers.
• **Continue for a minute or two.**

2 Then, stroke all around the crown of your baby's head in a circular direction using the relaxed weight of your palm and fingers.
• **Continue lightly for a minute or two.**

3 Now, using the relaxed weight of your whole hand, stroke all around the back of your baby's head, using a circular motion.
• **Continue for about a minute.**

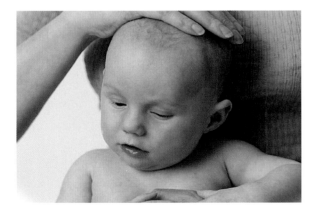

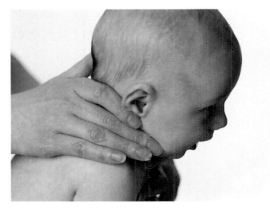

4 Continue the movement to include all of your baby's head. Stroke from the back of his head to the brow and around the crown.
• **Continue for as long as you like.**

5 Now stroke down the back of your baby's neck and shoulders and gently massage the back of his neck with your fingertips.
• **Continue for a minute or two**

If you use oil for this massage, make sure that you wipe your baby's brow to prevent the oil from entering his eyes, as it may temporarily blur his vision. (Used regularly, olive oil can be effective for treating cradle cap.)

Toe-to-Top Massage

CRANIOSACRAL TECHNIQUE

At two months, your baby's arms and legs are beginning to straighten and at three months she can stretch out her limbs more easily. If your baby is very fractious and has had a difficult delivery, long labor, or needed forceps or ventouse, you will be able to help her relax through her neck and shoulders. Unlike the toe-to-top full-body massage, this routine begins at the head (cranium) and moves down through the back (and to the sacrum). This is because the emphasis here is on physical alignment of the head and neck and relaxation of the neck and shoulders. Relieving pain and tension in this area will help your baby be far less fractious. The neck is

another emotional area and many things can be a "pain in the neck"; a long, difficult labor is certainly one of these as far as your baby is concerned.

You need to choose the right moment for this technique—the best time may be just after the full massage routine, when your baby is completely relaxed and happy, or after your baby has had her bath—when she is at her least active. You also will need your partner or a friend to perform the entire technique.

CRANIOSACRAL THERAPY
The key to this manipulative therapy is the lightness of the touch and the gentle alignment of the head and neck.

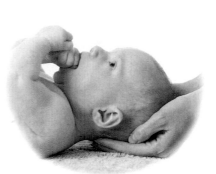

1 Lay your baby gently on her back in front of you, with the crown of her head towards you. Sit behind her and, with your hands open and relaxed, slip your palms under the base of your baby's head and rest them on the floor like a pillow.

2 Gently position your baby's head so that it is perfectly centerd, with her chin tucked into her chest to relax and lengthen the back of her neck. Hold your baby's head in this way for about a minute.

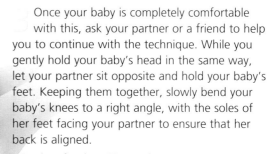

Once your baby is completely comfortable with this, ask your partner or a friend to help you to continue with the technique. While you gently hold your baby's head in the same way, let your partner sit opposite and hold your baby's feet. Keeping them together, slowly bend your baby's knees to a right angle, with the soles of her feet facing your partner to ensure that her back is aligned.

• **Continue for about 20 seconds.**

4 Keep holding your baby's head as your partner gently shakes your baby's legs straight before stroking them lightly down the front from her hips to her feet. Let your partner talk, sing and kiss your baby to fully engage her as he does this.

• **Continue for about 20 seconds.**

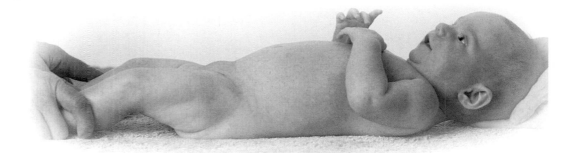

3 SECURING YOUR BABY'S POSTURE

The stages of motor development are universal and like the development of intelligence, each stage depends upon achieving the previous one. For example, your baby must sit before he can stand and stand before he can walk and so forth. The age at which he sits, crawls, stands and walks has no bearing upon his intellectual potential and each child, being unique, does this in his or her own time. Some babies sit late and walk early while others sit early and walk late.

Sitting properly is an art, a major accomplishment for all young babies, and like all the other stages of development, your baby should not be pushed into it nor hurried through it. There is no prescriptive time span on sitting, so take your cues from your baby. Your aim is to help him to secure this part of his development—to massage him through it so that he has the healthiest and most comfortable posture he could wish for.

Continuing to massage your baby can become a challenge once he is sitting on his own. He may no longer be content to lie down for his massage now that he has achieved this stage of development. You will need to work with him to accommodate his changing positions so that he continues to reap the benefits of a comprehensive massage.

Key benefits of seated massage

- Accomplishes a comfortable and healthy posture.

- Maintains abdominal breathing.

- Aids digestion.

- Promotes free and easy movement of the spine in all forward directions.

- Consolidates your baby's posture and helps him to develop confidence in sitting alone.

- Enables you to accommodate your baby's increasing mobility by modifying your techniques.

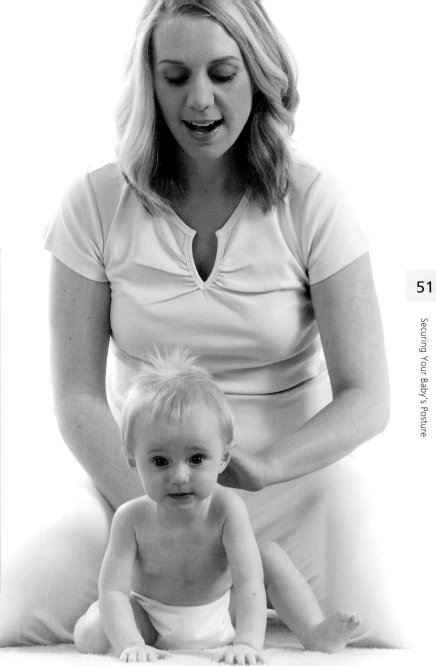

Helping Your Baby to Sit

During his early weeks, your baby has little strength to support his head and neck and any attempts to pull him up into a sitting position before he is ready will result in him dropping his head forwards and rounding his back. This is an uncomfortable and unhealthy posture, which weakens his spine and can inhibit breathing and digestion, so it is best avoided.

By two to three months, your baby should have developed the neck and shoulder strength to begin to work towards a healthy sitting posture. When he is able to lay on his belly with his head held up in line with his chest, he is ready to start the preliminary stage of sitting—with your help.

To sit comfortably for any period of time, your baby's hip joints must be flexible enough to allow him to sit on the back of his legs leaning forwards. This position enables free movement of the spine in all forward directions. It also permits his chest to remain open to accommodate a deeper breathing rhythm and his belly to remain relaxed so as not to inhibit the rhythms of digestion.

Do not pull your baby into a sitting position by his hands. His wrists do not form properly for some years and this will increase the curvature of your baby's back.

STRONG STRAIGHT BACK
Sitting up supported by a strong, straight back will enable your baby to accomplish many new skills and is a major step towards

1 Sit your baby up—with his feet together and his knees open (this is known as "tailor pose"). Kneel behind him and slip your left hand around his chest so that he can lean forwards into your palm for support, while taking his weight on the backs of his legs.

2 Now, with the fingertips of your right hand, gently stroke the crown of your baby's head to relax him.

• Continue for about 20 seconds.

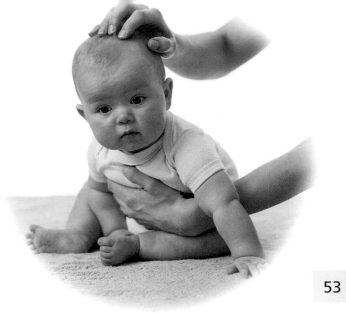

3 Relax your hand, and, using your palm, massage gently all around the crown and sides of his head.

• Continue for about 20 seconds.

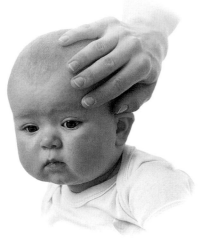

4 Stroke down your baby's back from the back of his head to the base of his spine with the weight of your relaxed hand. This will encourage him to transfer his weight downwards onto the backs of his thighs, which in turn will elongate his back for a healthy posture.

• Continue for about 20 seconds.

53

Securing Your Baby's Posture

Sitting Supported

Your baby will gain strength spending some waking time in the belly-forwards position, and you will know when he is ready to progress to sitting alone (from relying on you for this) when he can lay on his belly and support himself on his forearms and hands.

If he tries to sit unsupported at this stage, he could fall backwards, forwards over his feet or sideways, so you need to make sure that he is supported from all sides.

Sit him in the "tailor pose" sitting position—his feet should be together and his knees open. Lean him forwards over a long pillow or cushion placed over his legs, and place a cushion on each side to enclose him in a triangle. The emphasis is on his leaning forwards so that he can push himself up straight so ensure that he is sitting well— on the backs of his legs.

Never leave your baby unattended when he is sitting up with the support of cushions.

SAFE SURROUNDINGS
Make sure that your baby is completely surrounded by padding as he sits in the tailor pose.

1 Once your baby can support himself, take away the surrounding cushions and let him lean forwards so that he is supporting his trunk on straight arms, for as long as he is comfortable. Support him by holding him lightly around the waist or hips.

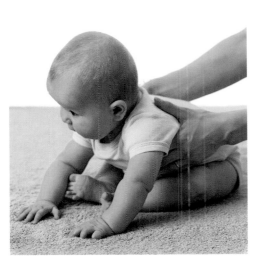

2 Now withdraw support from his back by moving your hands downwards and resting your relaxed hands over your baby's legs to "ground" him as he gets his balance. Leave his arms free to support himself.

3 Keep practicing this until you feel that your baby is confident and secure in this position; then you can begin to include massage. Steady him with one hand and massage downwards on the back of his hips with your other hand to help him secure his balance.

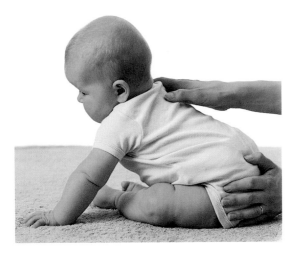

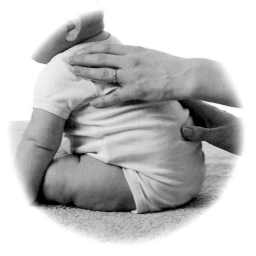

4 Follow this by massaging hand over hand down his back from his shoulders to his lower back, still gently pushing the back of his hips and the base of his spine downwards.

Sitting Unsupported

Sitting unsupported is usually achieved around six or seven months of age. When your baby is fully secure with sitting on her own, she will be able to reach for her favorite toys, take a cup or cracker and stretch her arms up to you to be lifted. Massage here can help your baby to strengthen and consolidate her posture and to develop more confidence while sitting independently. You can modify some of the techniques for your baby now that she is able to sit without your support and concentrate on those that will benefit her the most at this stage of her development.

This is an important time for your baby, so don't hurry her onto the crawling stage. Practice will help her to perfect these postures and she is developing the skills that will last her a lifetime. She will know when she has practiced enough to move on.

EXTRA SUPPORT
By kneeling with your baby in between your legs, you can offer her support—should she require it—as she learns to sit alone.

1 As your baby sits, kneel behind her and stroke down her back, hand-over-hand, and around the hips and tops of her legs.

• **Continue for about 20 seconds.**

3 Now, provided that your baby's belly is not full, massage her tummy from side to side, by kneading gently with a cupped hand between the ribs and the hips.

• **Continue for about 20 seconds.**

2 Stroke over her shoulders and gently pull her arms through your relaxed palms downwards and sideways. This will help relax her arms and shoulders in this position. You may want to use oil here, so that your hands glide easily and you do not pull her off balance.

• **Continue for about 20 seconds.**

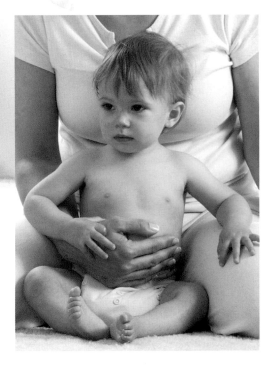

Sitting Japanese-Style

When your baby has fully secured the tailor pose and is ready to move onto all fours, he will lean forwards over his feet and then pull himself forwards onto his hands and knees. He may spend some time pulling forwards and then rocking back into the tailor pose, but soon he will bring his knees together and then sit back between his feet—a traditionally Japanese position. This is an easy foundation for making the transition from sitting to crawling and your baby may now start to prefer this position to the tailor pose.

You will have to choose the right moment to massage your baby once he is in this position, because once he gets mobile, he will not want to remain still for long.

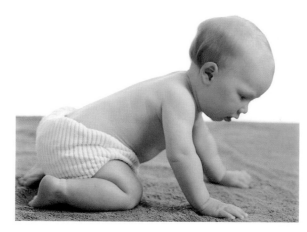

FIXING THE FEET
Some babies sit in this posture with their feet turned outwards. If you notice your baby doing this, correct it by gently turning the feet inwards—a much healthier position for his knees and hips.

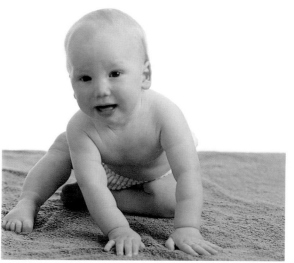

1 Sitting behind your baby, massage the front of his thighs—from the knees to the hips—stroking backwards and forwards with oiled, relaxed hands. This will relax his front thighs.

• **Continue for about 20 seconds.**

2 Now try to encourage your baby to lean back towards you at about a 30 degree angle. This will help to further relax the front of his thighs and will keep his lower back straight and strong.

• **Continue for about 20 seconds.**

3 Let your baby sit up straight again. Cup your hand slightly and, to relax your baby's belly, stroke from right to left with a circular movement. This can also aid his digestion.

• **Continue for about 20 seconds.**

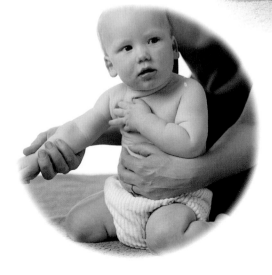

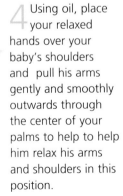

4 Using oil, place your relaxed hands over your baby's shoulders and pull his arms gently and smoothly outwards through the center of your palms to help to help him relax his arms and shoulders in this position.

• **Continue for about 20 seconds.**

Securing Your Baby's Posture

4

MOBILITY AND SOFT GYMNASTICS

Once your baby is able to sit independently, he will begin moving out of his first sitting position. As he moves from sitting to crawling, he will develop his second sitting position and go on to squat, stand and walk. Having created a wide range of versatile movements, your baby will now start to strengthen rapidly and in carrying and moving his ever-increasing body weight from place to place, he will become a little "weight lifter." The more body weight he lifts, the stronger your baby will become and, like all weight lifters, unless he continues to make expansive movements, he will lose some of his flexibility as he strengthens.

As your baby starts to crawl, squat, stand and walk, he will no longer wish to stay still for a structured massage, but the following soft gymnastic techniques allow you to continue to positively influence his development while he is on the move. They can be used for fun and games while maintaining good posture and all-round structural fitness as your baby grows. And they will enable you to continue engaging your baby on a one-to-one basis, to share lots of love and affection.

Like massage, these soft gymnastic games should never be forced or practiced against your child's will, and you do not have to do all of the stretches in one go. It is better to try them one at a time until you are completely confident and your baby anticipates and enjoys them. You can then aim to fit them in once or twice a week.

Key benefits of soft gymnastics

- Encourage your baby to develop and maintain suppleness, good muscle tone and joint flexibility.

- Encourage your baby to develop and maintain an open chest and shoulders, a strong back and good posture as he grows and strengthens.

- Build up self-confidence and a good body image.

- Encourage structural symmetry and balance.

- Encourage your baby to maintain and develop abdominal breathing and muscular relaxation, both at rest and while in action.

- Encourage a more confident physical and emotional relationship with parents.

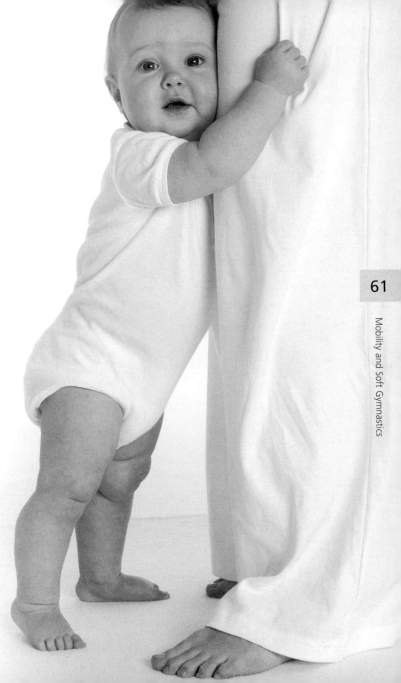

ENCOURAGING MOBILITY

Although most babies will crawl for some time before they stand and walk properly, some stand and walk without crawling. Usually, if a baby misses the crawling phase it is because he has not spent enough waking time laying on his tummy and is more reticent about moving onto all fours. Such babies are often "bottom shufflers," and will move themselves around—quite effectively—in a sitting position.

Babies that are used to laying on their bellies, once they are ready to begin crawling, will pull themselves forwards from the first sitting position—tailor pose—onto all fours. From here, first attempts at crawling often result in a baby moving backwards and, after some practice, he will begin to pull himself forwards using his arms and hands. After this, he usually begins to crawl on his hands and knees, but some babies crawl on their hands and feet.

At the same time as your baby makes his early attempts at crawling, he will develop his second sitting position and may begin to stand with support. As he develops strength and confidence, he will start to pull himself up from squatting to standing, with support, and practice lifting his legs. Once he is able to lift and lower one leg at a time, he will begin to enjoy walking sideways around furniture, and walking forwards holding your hands.

Walking

Once your baby is standing, you can encourage him to walk. Sit on the floor, opposite your partner—you should be close enough to touch each other's outstretched hands. With your baby standing in between you, call his name to encourage him to walk between you.

• **Continue for as long as you and your baby are having fun.**

63

Preparing

Once your baby is sitting independently, kneel on the floor and sit him over your thigh. Let him squat and stand with his feet either side of your thigh. This position keeps his hips, knees and ankles in line to encourage postural symmetry.

• **Continue for as long as you and your baby are comfortable.**

Crawling

To encourage your baby to crawl, rock him to and fro over your thigh, while he is in an all-fours position.

• **Continue for as long as you and your baby are comfortable.**

Standing

Stand him on his feet and hold him by the waist. Bear down gently, giving him the weight of your hands for stronger roots and better balance. You can develop this by taking your hands to his thighs and bearing down.

• **Continue for as long as it's fun and your baby is comfortable.**

Mobility and Soft Gymnastics

Tailor Pose Swing

When most adults sit on the floor, they tend to curve their spines and their weight is supported by their lower backs. This sitting position is not only uncomfortable to maintain for any length of time, but it is also damaging to the back and the spine and can inhibit the functions of breathing and digestion.

By practicing this technique, your baby will achieve the strength and flexibility necessary to enable him to continue to sit with his weight on the back of his thighs. This takes the strain off his lower back and maintains good sitting posture. Your baby's internal organs also benefit because in this position his chest is open and his tummy is relaxed, allowing him to breathe more deeply and encouraging a more healthy digestive rhythm.

This position is also practical for your developing baby—by maintaining flexibility, his spine is free to bend from his hip joints, allowing him to reach forwards freely in all directions.

As your baby progresses from sitting to standing, he may lose some of his flexibility and with it, his perfect sitting posture. It is important, therefore, to keep using the tailor pose swing to ensure that your child's hips remain flexible and that he retains a strong, straight back and good posture as he grows and develops.

The swing will soon become a game that your child will actively enjoy and look forward to—you may find that if you forget to do it, he will be quick to remind you.

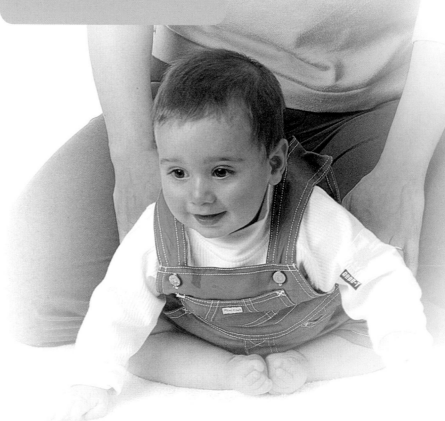

A NATURAL POSE
This is your baby's first sitting position. With his feet together and knees open, his legs and hips are in perfect symmetry.

1 Sit your baby on your lap in tailor pose with your arms under his arms and over his legs. Bring the soles of his feet together and gently pull them into the trunk of his body. Clap his feet together and slowly rock your baby from side to side.

• **Continue for about 20 seconds.**

2 Now raise yourself off your heels and support your baby by holding his ankles. Your baby will be held securely between your forearms.

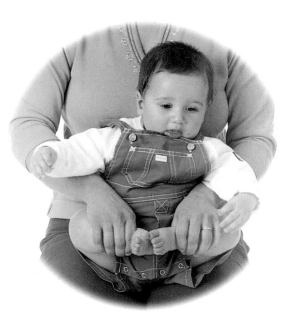

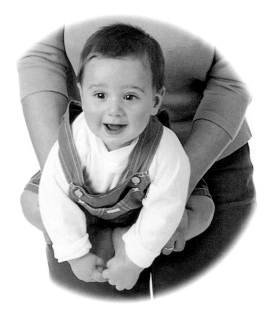

Throughout this soft gymnastic game, make sure that your arms remain under your baby's arms and over his legs.

3 Now start to swing your baby gently from side to side. Do this five or six times—as your baby finds his rhythm he will relax and begin to enjoy it. Continue to swing and now let your baby lean forwards, taking his chest towards his feet. Make sure that your arms remain under your baby's arms throughout the exercise.

• **Continue for 4–5 swings.**

65

Mobility and Soft Gymnastics

Strong, Flexible Legs

As the "roots" of the body, the legs must be strong enough to support and carry it and supple enough to allow a wide range of movement from sitting and standing, to jumping and running. When your baby begins to explore his range of movement and "finds his feet," he will become more confident and a little more independent.

As your baby's legs strengthen, he will no longer stand and walk with his legs and feet open "cowboy style" because his inside thigh muscles will contract and draw them in line with his hips. At the same time, other postural muscles—such as in the calves, front thighs and buttocks—will strengthen to make his legs more stable. If these muscles strengthen without being stretched, your baby can lose a degree of his body's range of movement. For example, he will no longer be able to take his foot to his face or enjoy the freedom of movement in tailor pose.

Your baby has spent a great deal of time and effort establishing a wide range of movement and it makes good sense to help him to retain this as he gains strength. Playing these soft gymnastic games once or twice a week will ensure that your baby maintains flexible joints and continues to enjoy a wide variety of movement and good posture.

KEEPING HIPS FLEXIBLE
You can help to maintain the flexibility of your baby's hips by sitting with him so that his legs are outstretched around your waist.

1 Sit your baby on your thighs and lean back slightly as you take your baby's feet to his face. Rock him from side to side and sing to him.

• **Continue for about half a minute.**

2 Hold one of your baby's legs from the back of the thigh and knee, and let the other leg straighten. Rub and massage the back of the thigh as you continue to rock and sing.

• **Continue for half a minute. Repeat with his other leg.**

3 Let your baby sit between your knees in "side-splits"—with his legs and feet open. Close one leg in a half tailor pose, then straighten it and close the other.

• **Repeat this movement from leg to leg rhythmically for about half a minute.**

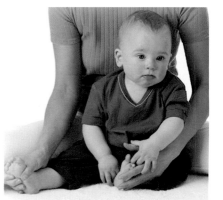

4 As your baby sits upright, open both of his legs. Rock him while you gently massage his inner thighs.

• **Continue for 20–30 seconds.**

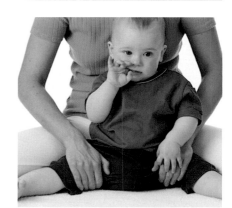

5 Gently bring your baby's legs together and, keeping his legs straight, extend his heels by taking his feet in your hands then turning them out.

• **Hold for a few seconds.**

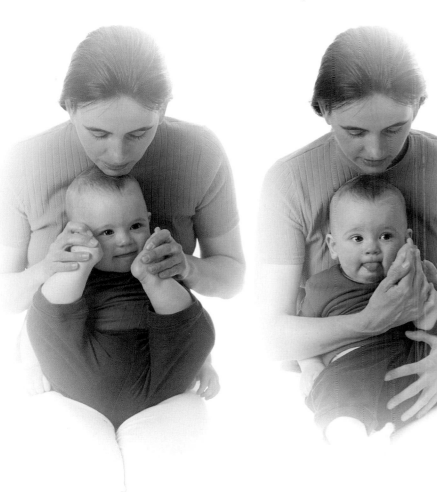

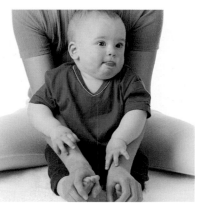

Mobility and Soft Gymnastics

An Open Chest and Shoulders

Unlike adults, who usually restrict their breathing to their chests and inhibit their emotional expressions to facial and hand movements, the child expresses herself with her whole body—jumping up and down and throwing open her arms with delight or shaking her fists and stamping her feet with rage. Babies are active; their responses are spontaneous and their breathing rhythm is full and easy.

Young children have an intuitive understanding of the intimate relationship between feeling, breathing and movement. As well as expressing their emotions with uninhibited movement, to suppress feeling—to subdue fear or acute anxiety—they will make themselves motionless, become very still and hold their breath.

Observe how your baby sits and stands; her straight back, free chest and relaxed shoulders reveal a positive attitude to life and a state of mind untainted by negativity. Watch how your baby breathes; every breath descends deep into her belly and her chest and abdomen work in harmony—expanding and contracting together.

Your baby's straight back and her open chest and shoulders illustrate the structural balance of her posture, where weight is easily carried and transferred bone upon bone without undue stress being placed upon the muscles. This allows the muscles to function healthily and to retain a high degree of relaxation even when the body is mobile.

Even from an early age, babies enjoy arching their backs and it is this intuitive movement that contributes greatly to the healthy nature of theirs posture and breathing rhythms.

DOUBLY BENEFICIAL
This exercise encourages full relaxation throughout the front of your baby's body and strengthens her back and spine.

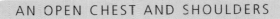

2 Now let your baby lay back over your thighs, so that her feet remain on the floor and her head and back are arched. To encourage this movement, rock your baby gently and slowly roll your legs from side to side while you sing to her.

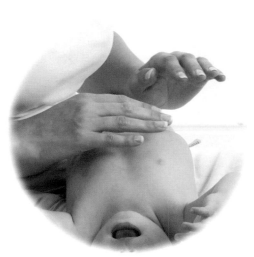

3 Once your baby is relaxed in this position, pat her chest with cupped hands, rub her belly clockwise and stroke down the front of her thighs. Keep rolling your legs gently as you continue this light massage.

• **Continue for about half a minute.**

1 Sit on the floor against a wall or on the edge of a cushion with your legs straight. When you are comfortable, sit your baby across your lap, so that she is facing to one side.

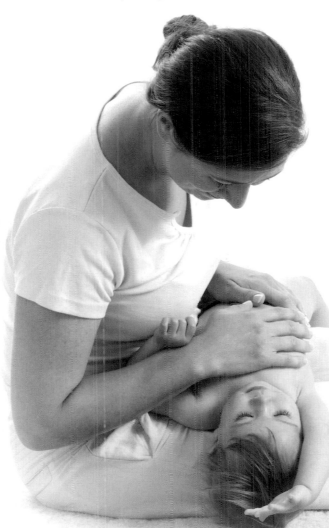

Your baby will soon learn to anticipate backbending and will lay back more readily and remain a little longer in this position while you rub her tummy, chest and shoulders.

69

Mobility and Soft Gymnastics

Back Strength and Flexibility

Children constantly engage in vigorous physical games and activities that often demand a wide range of physical movement. The flexibility of the spine and the strength of the muscles that support it are therefore of great importance.

Once he can stand, your child must secure his balance and will continually test the boundaries of his movements and the potential abilities of his body. This will undoubtedly involve the odd tumble or two, but because children are more relaxed than adults—both in action and at rest—the shock of impact when they fall generally passes right through their bodies.

You can engage your baby in the following soft gymnastic game once he is on his feet and continue for as long as you can lift him and you both enjoy it. Practiced once or twice a week, it will help to maintain and improve your child's suppleness throughout the front of his body, the overall flexibility of his spine and the strength of his back. It is also of great benefit to your baby's posture and promotes all the physiological benefits of good health and the self-confidence that accompanies fitness and good posture.

DUAL PURPOSE ACTIVITY
This is also a trust game and one in which your baby's world turns upside-down and then he centers himself.

1 Kneeling comfortably on your feet, on a cushion, sit your baby on your lap, facing you, belly to belly.

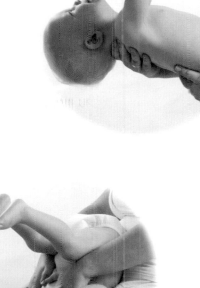

2 Now, holding his legs securely around the sides of your body under your arms, place both of your hands on his back—one at the base of his neck, the other around his lower back, across his hips. Let your baby lean backwards and gently open his chest and shoulders by pushing his upper back. Talk, sing and rock him gently, keeping him fully engaged.

• **Continue for about 20 seconds.**

3 Now, lower your baby and let him lean back over your knees, and place your hands over his shoulders. Rock your thighs gently from side to side to relax your baby.

• **Continue for about 20 seconds.**

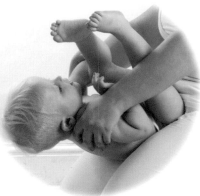

4 Your hands must be on the insides of your baby's arms. Making sure that your baby's legs can roll unimpeded, stand up on your knees, supporting him from over his shoulders, and let him roll backwards through your arms.

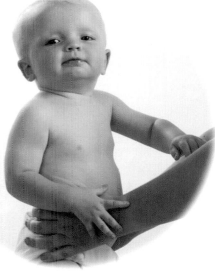

5 When he has landed in a standing position, drop your hands down, hold him from around the hips and bear down gently using just the weight of your hands to "ground" him.

Mobility and Soft Gymnastics

REINTRODUCING MASSAGE

Increasing mobility and the urge to explore generally mean that most babies go through a period during which they resist laying still long enough for an "all over" massage. When this happens, don't undress your baby for massage, but whenever you are sitting together, continue to rub her back and her head, arms, legs and feet. Try to maintain this kind of affectionate touch whenever it is mutually enjoyable. Although your baby may not want to be undressed and massaged, the need to be held and touched is still tremendously important; your sustained physical reassurances will continue to add to your child's sense of self-worth and her healthy body image. Lots of spontaneous hugs, kisses and strokes will add to your baby's self-esteem and will make it easier for you to reintroduce massage into your relationship. When you feel the time is right, usually around 18 months, try to introduce the following routine in your child's time rather than yours. This is usually when she is at her most relaxed—before her afternoon nap or before she goes to bed, for example—but not on an empty or full tummy.

CONTINUED CLOSENESS
The need to be held and touched continues throughout life.
Maintain enjoyable physical contact with your child as she grows
and develops.

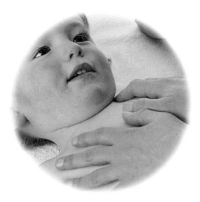

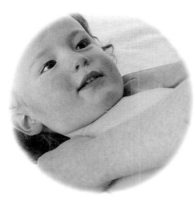

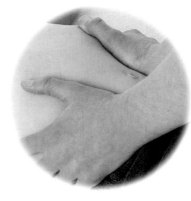

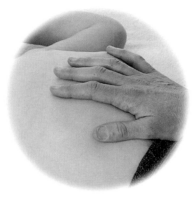

1 Place both hands on the center of your child's chest and massage upwards, outwards and back to the center with your relaxed hands.

• **Repeat 4–5 times.**

2 Rub your child's shoulders gently but firmly, backwards and forwards from the sides of his neck outwards.

• **Continue for about 20 seconds.**

3 Keeping your hands on your child's skin, stroke downwards from the shoulders to the hips and back again.

• **Repeat 4–5 times.**

4 Using the relaxed weight of one hand, massage your child's belly clockwise in a circular motion.

• **Repeat 5–6 times.**

73

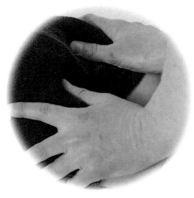

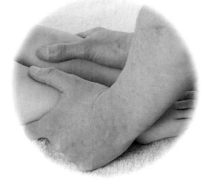

5 Massage the front of your child's thighs by squeezing and releasing and rubbing gently five or six times then slide your hands to his calves and repeat the movements.

6 Keep your hands on your child's skin and stroke back up to his shoulders and right down to his feet.

• **Repeat 3–4 times, ending with the feet.**

Mobility and Soft Gymnastics

A stronger touch

The onset of the "terrible twos," from about 18 months, is the time your baby begins to assert herself and her quest for independence, and requires even more patience and understanding on your part. Appropriately, it seems that around this age there are periods when babies once again enjoy being massaged and these interludes can often provide a welcome break in the emotional extremes that may prevail at this time.

Now that your baby is stronger and more resilient, you may need to add more depth to your touch and give a slightly stronger and faster massage. To keep your baby's attention, you must continue to talk, sing and maintain eye-contact with your child as much as you can, for as long as you massage. If you have been practicing the soft gymnastic games on pages 60–71, you may wish to combine massage with one or two of them. Take opportunities as well to air-bathe your baby as she enjoys her mobility.

BENEFICIAL COMBINATION
Use the soft gymnastic games combined with massage as a means of setting your bay on the road to independence.

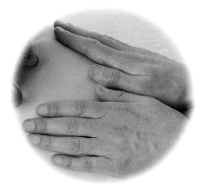

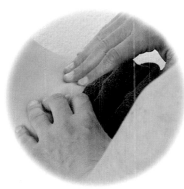

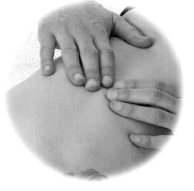

9 With the middle fingers and index fingers of both hands, glide up both sides of your baby's back from the base of the spine to the back of the neck and back down again.

• **Continue for about 20 seconds.**

7 With your baby laying on his belly, rub his shoulders with your palms and massage the sides of his upper spine, pressing in gently with your thumbs.

• **Continue for about 20 seconds.**

8 Stroke down your baby's back from his shoulders to his feet, using the relaxed weight of both hands. Using your fingertips, massage the base of his spine and rub gently.

• **Repeat 3–4 times.**

11 To finish, stroke down the back of your baby's body from shoulders to feet.

• **Repeat 3–4 times.**

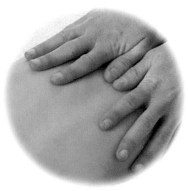

10 Now spread your fingers and draw the relaxed weight of your hands all the way down to the feet. Glide your hands back up to the base of your baby's spine.

• **Repeat 3–4 times.**

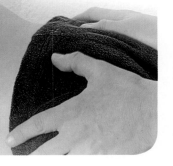

Mobility and Soft Gymnastics

5

THERAPEUTIC TOUCH FOR SICKNESS AND ADDITIONAL NEEDS

Many childhood ailments and illnesses render the skin hypersensitive and "prickly" and when your baby is distinctly unwell, she will not want to be massaged in the normal way. Quite often what a baby most wants and needs is to sleep and be held until the prescribed remedy becomes effective. In instances like this, when you find yourself lying or sitting comfortably with your baby, try gently squeezing and kneading her hands and feet and stroking her head lightly with your fingertips—these

If your baby shows symptoms of illness, such as a high temperature, listlessness and irritability, watery eyes or runny nose, always seek professional advice—a prompt diagnosis can hasten your baby's recovery.

techniques are non-invasive and can be relaxing and comforting.

The same approach can be used if your baby is emotionally upset, if she does not respond well to touch, finds it difficult to relax and let go when being held, and cries easily.

In the following chapter are some techniques for more specific conditions, but none of these are meant to be used as a substitute for professional diagnosis and recommendations.

Babies with additional needs can also benefit from massage and you can modify techniques or bring out certain elements of massage to suit particular needs.

Key benefits of therapeutic touch techniques

- Soothe common childhood complaints.

- Can comfort a generally fractious child.

- Help you to combat various types of congestion.

- Enable parents to ease physical problems.

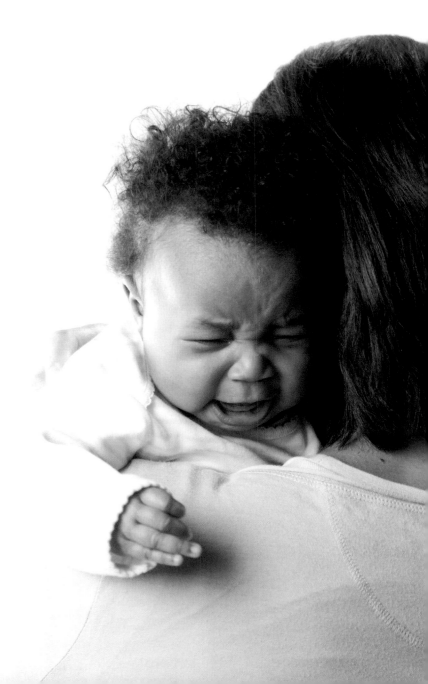

Coughs, Colds and Congestion

A young baby will only breathe through his mouth when his nostrils are completely blocked with mucus. In the daytime, this may not cause too much of a problem, but at night it can prove to be a major source of discomfort. When your baby sleeps, his breathing rhythm becomes slower and deeper and if his nostrils are congested, he will gasp for air and awake with a start. This can be quite disruptive, particularly if your baby has already established a sleeping routine.

If your baby is congested, place him in a more upright position when he is sleeping. You can do this by raising one end of his cot by securely placing a book or telephone directory underneath—don't let your baby sleep on a pillow. And avoid giving him mucus-making foods, such as dairy products.

These techniques will show you how to relieve nostril and chest congestion, but they are not meant as a substitute for a professional diagnosis and treatment, rather as an aid to your baby's recovery. You may want to try the technique for freeing blocked nostrils on yourself first before using it on your baby.

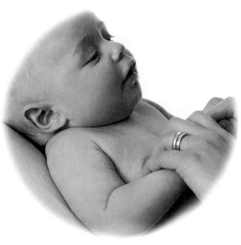

1 Sit on the floor with your back resting against a wall and your knees raised. Put your baby on your lap so that he is facing you.

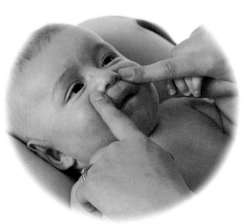

2 Gently press your index fingertips into each side of your baby's nostrils and draw the nostrils open by pressing gently downwards and outwards under the cheekbones.

• **Repeat 4–5 times.**

EASING CHEST CONGESTION

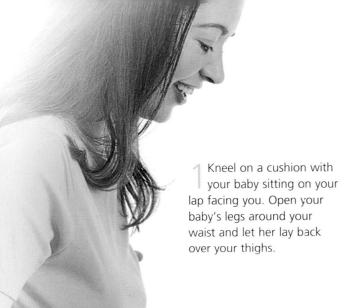

1 Kneel on a cushion with your baby sitting on your lap facing you. Open your baby's legs around your waist and let her lay back over your thighs.

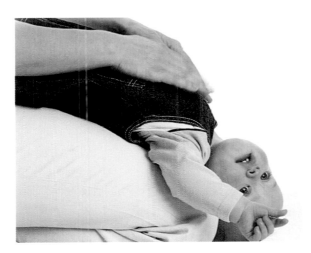

2 Using the relaxed weight of your cupped hands, pat all around the center, and then the sides, of your baby's chest.

• **Continue for about half a minute.**

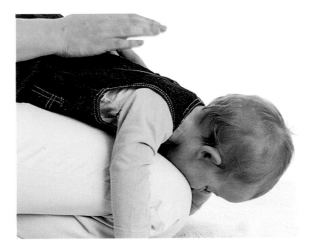

3 Now, place your baby on your thighs so she lays forwards on her belly and, using the relaxed weight of your cupped hands, pat all around her back and sides. If your baby is heavily congested, she may vomit slightly following this percussion movement, as the bronchial tubes compress and expel the mucus.

• **Continue for about half a minute.**

Some essential oils, such as eucalyptus and lavender, are recommended for clearing the sinuses. Mix 2–3 drops into your base oil. Do not use essential oils for babies under 10 weeks. Eucalyptus will cancel any benefits of homeopathic treatment.

Relieving Sticky Eye

It is not uncommon for babies to have sticky eyes in the first day or two of life—usually as a result of amniotic fluid and other secretions entering the eyes at birth—and this stickiness usually disappears spontaneously. Beyond the first 48 hours, however, a sticky eye is due to infection. Otherwise known as conjunctivitis, a red and sticky eye often clears if you cleanse the eye with a cotton wool swab and some tepid boiled water—gently wiping outwards from the inside corners. If redness and stickiness persist, medical advice should be sought.

An eye that is continuously sticky and watery can be due to a blocked tear duct. The tear ducts are lined with mucous membrane, an extension of that which lines the nostrils. When this membrane becomes inflamed and swollen, the tear ducts become blocked, causing tears to flow from the eyes rather than drain into the nose as they usually do. Try this simple technique to clear the blockage.

> Do not use oil for this technique as it can enter your baby's eye. Make sure that your hands are clean and that your fingernails cannot scratch your baby.

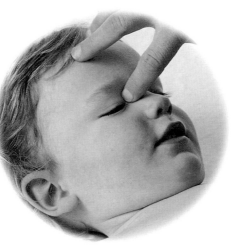

1 The tear glands and ducts are located in the depression in the nasal bone in the corner of the eye and run down the side of the bridge of the nose. Place your index finger outside the corner of your baby's eye and press gently into the side of the nose. You may need to steady your baby's head with your free hand while you do this.

2 Draw your finger downwards, along the side of your baby's nostril and under the cheekbone.

• Repeat 3–4 times.

Treating Glue Ear

If your baby has any ear discharge, other than wax, or appears to be in pain, consult your doctor immediately. This could be a middle ear infection that needs immediate medical attention.

Glue ear refers to the discharge of a thick, sticky substance in the middle ear, which prevents the eardrum from moving normally and can cause partial deafness. This chronic condition is often the result of recurrent episodes of acute otitis media (middle ear infection).

Glue ear can sometimes be treated by a competent cranial osteopath but, as a preventive measure, try the following sequence when you massage your baby's head and neck. You may wish to use some oil to make the movement smoother.

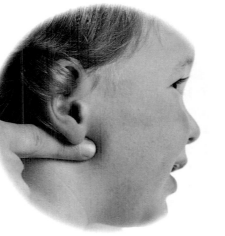

2 Press your fingers gently into the sides of your baby's upper jawbone, behind his ears, and draw them downwards around the edge of the jawbone towards his throat.

• **Repeat 3–4 times.**

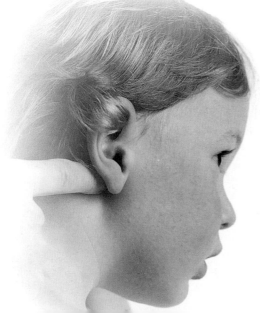

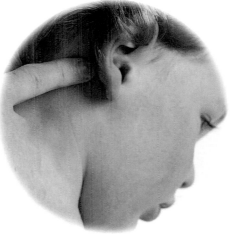

1 With your baby facing away from you, place your index fingers on the side of his head, behind the lobes of his ears.

3 Now, press your index fingers again behind the lobes of both of your baby's ears and gently draw them downwards and towards you, around the sides and base of the skull.

• **Repeat 3–4 times.**

Wind, Colic and Constipation

We all take in air while we are eating and drinking, but because of the immaturity of your young baby's digestive system, air in the stomach or intestines can result in an uncomfortable pocket of gas. Wind is more common in bottle-fed babies so the first thing to check is that the hole in the teat is neither too small nor too large—the formula should drip out at a steady flow of one drop per second. Also ensure that the bottle is tilted and that the milk completely fills the teat. Both situations will result in your baby taking in too much air with his milk. Try to keep your baby's back straight while feeding and when he has finished, pat him between the shoulder blades and stroke his back upwards from the bottom to the top, while tilting him forwards slightly.

No one really knows what causes colic—long spells of crying that usually occur at night—and there are no certain cures, but if you are breastfeeding; eating wholesome, nourishing foods regularly and giving yourself time to eat properly, these may help. It is also not uncommon for breastfed babies to go for a few days occasionally without emptying their bowels. Giving your baby plenty of waking time on his belly (see page 18) can prevent and relieve reflux, colic and constipation as this position stretches and relaxes the abdomen, but do not do this immediately after a feed—let him digest his food first.

You also can use tummy massage but not when your baby is distressed—try Tiger in the Tree (see page 88) instead. The following technique can be used between bouts of discomfort, when your baby is neither too hungry nor too full. A good opportunity for this massage is when you are changing your baby's nappy.

SOFTEN THE BELLY
If your baby's belly is hard and unyielding, gently move his hands out of the way then gently lay your relaxed hand across the belly before you begin to massage.

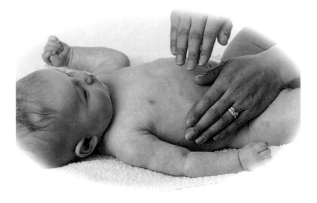 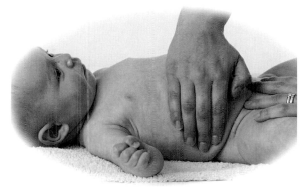

If your baby is suffering from wind, colic or constipation, consult your doctor to rule out the possibility that your baby is allergic to something in his diet or, if you are breastfeeding, something in yours. If your baby has started on solids, try giving him pureed papaya fruit, which contains enzymes to aid his digestion.

1 Lay your baby on the floor and, using the relaxed weight of your whole hand, massage hand-over-hand down the right side of his abdomen, from between the hip and the lower rib across to below the navel.

• **Continue for 2–3 minutes and then repeat on the left side of your baby's abdomen.**

2 Cup your hand and place it horizontally across your baby's belly. Squeeze gently and knead the belly from side to side. Don't push downwards or your baby will resist and tense up. Keep it gentle and playful, so that his belly softens.

• **Continue for about 20 seconds**

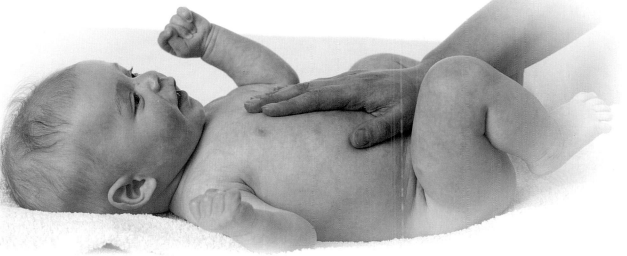

3 Now, using the relaxed weight of your cupped hand, massage your baby's belly with your hand and the tummy moving in a circular motion clockwise from your left to your right.

• **Repeat 4–5 times.**

Therapeutic Touch for Sickness and Additional Needs

Teething and Irritability

Teething starts some weeks before your baby's teeth make an appearance, which can be any time between three and 12 months. The first tooth is usually the lower central incisor and following this, other incisors appear—three up and three down, enabling your baby to bite. Altogether, your baby will cut 20 milk teeth—as opposed to 32 permanent teeth, which will start to appear when she is about six years of age.

Most teeth erupt without any detectable pain or discomfort but in the day or two before or after eruption, your baby may exhibit some fussiness, drooling and a desire to chomp on a hard object. If your baby suffers discomfort, a hard, cold object—such as a gel-filled teething ring—may provide relief. If your baby is experiencing particular distress, massaging her hands, feet and back is non-intrusive and can comfort her when she is restless and upset.

There are many symptoms incorrectly attributed to teething such as fever, diarrhea, poor appetite, vomiting, coughing and a runny nose. As any of these could be the result of a serious illness, if your baby appears to be unwell, seek professional advice.

SIGNS OF TEETHING
Some babies salivate and press their hands into their mouths when they are teething.

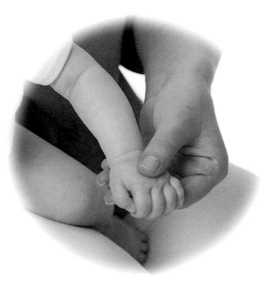

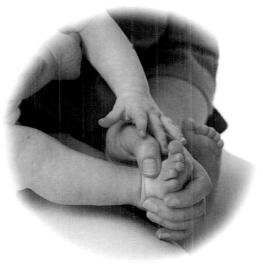

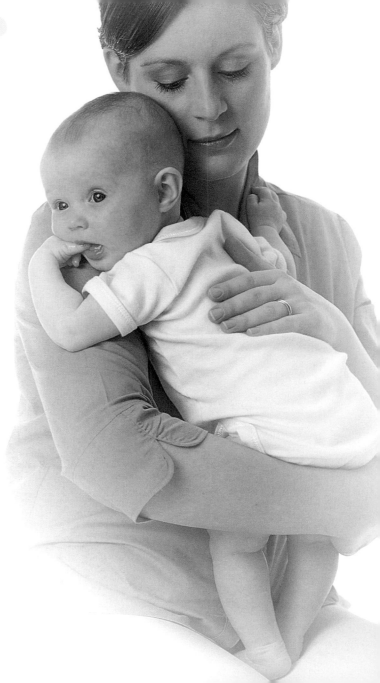

1 Sitting with your baby on your lap, squeeze and stroke her hands gently between your thumb and fingers.

2 Take the massage down to your baby's feet, squeezing gently and stroking both the tops and the soles of her feet.

A natural remedy such as chamomile roman can be effective for soothing your baby during teething. Dilute a few drops in full-fat milk and pour this into your baby's bath.

3 Now, hold your baby close and stroke her gently all over her back and up and down the length of her spine. Talk to her softly as you massage her.

Sleeplessness

Most young babies do not sleep through the night. Your baby has been close to you for nine months so to expect him to conform to a routine in a new and unfamiliar environment is unrealistic. A young baby needs feeding fairly often so your baby cannot help but interrupt your sleep to be fed. Once fed and changed, your baby should return to sleep after a cuddle. Remember that physical contact is as vital for babies, and a little

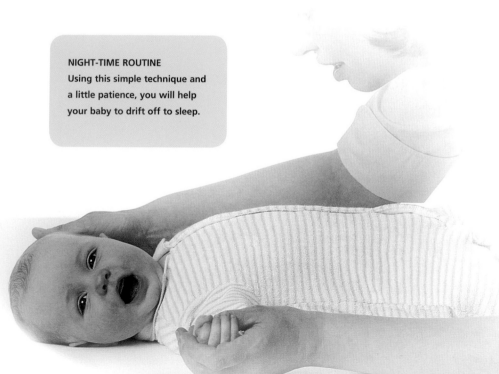

NIGHT-TIME ROUTINE
Using this simple technique and a little patience, you will help your baby to drift off to sleep.

time spent in your arms is often all that is needed for your baby settle. (Tiger in the Tree is deeply relaxing, see page 88.)

After your baby has settled into a longer sleep routine he may still resist going to bed and when awakened returning back to sleep. If your baby is not hungry or uncomfortable and stops crying while he is in your arms but cries when you try to lay him down, the following technique could be extremely useful. It will allow you to withdraw gradually, to offer your baby a loving touch that will reassure him of your presence and induce tranquillity and sleep.

Much of the success of this technique will depend upon you positioning yourself comfortably, persevering and being consistent. Once your baby has accepted it, you will find that the technique will induce sleep, and that your baby will begin to anticipate it.

The same technique can be used when you feel that the time is right to introduce a routine and put your baby to bed at a regular hour. You can begin to withdraw further by shortening the time spent stroking but leaving your hands on your baby until he is sleeping. When you have established this, you can reduce the time still further and remove your hands when your baby is almost asleep—but remain within sight of him and quietly reassure him. If your baby is able to sit and sits up crying, lay him down and continue. The final step is to lay your baby down, stroke him, tell him it's time to sleep and slowly withdraw.

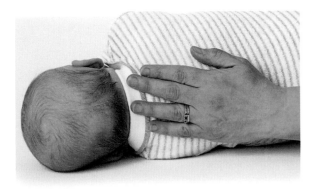

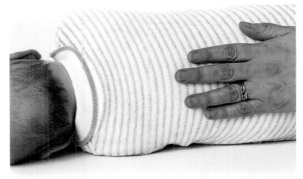

1 Start by laying your baby on his side; you can always turn him onto his back once he is asleep. Stroke around the top of his back or head using the relaxed weight of your whole hand.

2 Then stroke down the length of his back in the same way as you would a puppy or a kitten.

Always lay your baby down on his back to sleep. As he gets older, he may turn to his side and then onto his tummy but by then he'll be at a much lower risk of sudden infant death syndrome (SIDS).

87

3 Place a relaxed hand across your baby's head, which fits perfectly into the palm of your hand and your fingers.

4 Keeping one hand on your baby's head, place a relaxed hand across your baby's tummy and knead the tummy very gently from side to side. As your baby relaxes, this will induce feelings of tranquillity. Withdraw very slowly once your baby is sleeping.

• DO NOT LEAVE YOUR BABY TO "CRY IT OUT." Persevere with the technique as a crying baby separated from his mother has high levels of stress hormones and this is not good for babies (or for mothers).

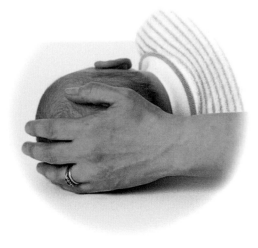

TIGER IN THE TREE

Tiger in the tree is a wonderful position in which you can hold and massage your baby from birth to relax her tummy and relieve birth trauma, colic, wind, constipation, fractiousness, anxiety and other ailments associated with acute abdominal tension.

The technique is both curative and preventative—it can be used on the spot to bring instant relief to your baby when she needs it most, as well as on a daily basis to help her develop a cumulative sense of ease that can dramatically improve her whole disposition. It does not succeed, however, if your baby is hungry.

The tummy is an emotional center and a great source of tranquillity. Keep your baby's tummy relaxed and you will keep your baby relaxed. Having her lay forwards in your arms, combined with gentle side-to-side abdominal massage, initiates a deep sense of relief and relaxation that pervades her entire body. Supporting your baby on both of your arms allows you to sustain the position for a longer period of time, so that your baby enjoys the maximum effect of the massage.

Fathers, especially, will find this is a useful technique because the baby is facing away from the breast and will not add to her discomfort by trying to feed. It also gives

them a successful position in which to soothe a distressed baby when a mother is absent or needs time to herself.

The way in which you hold and massage your baby is essential to the success of this technique. Maintain your own sense of relaxation by keeping your shoulders and hands relaxed and your breathing deep and rhythmic. Take your time and rock, talk or sing softly and your baby will sense your calmness and adapt to you, rather than you becoming upset and adapting to her.

This technique can be practiced with your baby naked or clothed. Its effects are immediate and it can be performed anywhere and at any time. Your baby does not need to be upset to practice this technique. Get her used to this position. The more you practice, the easier it gets and the greater the benefits.

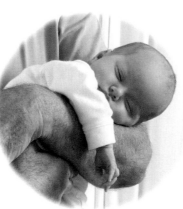

SLEEP AID
Your baby will probably fall asleep in your arms once her discomfort has been relieved by this technique.

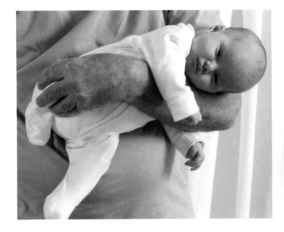

1 Hold your baby with her back to you and bring your left arm across your baby's chest, taking care to drop her left arm under yours so that you can comfortably cradle her head and neck in the crook of your elbow.

2 Bring your right hand between your baby's knees and place your palm across your baby's tummy, supporting her equally in both of your arms. Tuck your baby's foot into the crook of your arm and turn her over onto your hand.

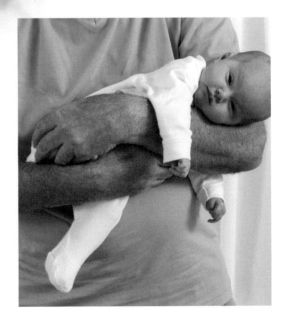

INTERNAL ORGANS

With your hand spread, your thumb is on the ascending colon and your fingers are on the descending colon (both between the lower ribs and hips).

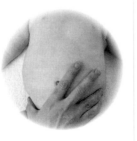

3 As she lies belly forwards over your hand, very gently knead her tummy from side to side with your relaxed hand. The weight of her body as it lies on your working hand adds to the efficiency of the massage as you are able to attain deeper contact without pressing in. If, after a few minutes, your baby continues to experience discomfort, walk her around in this position and gently pat her chest.

• **Repeat this technique frequently and try to establish the position as a regular holding position.**

Caesarean Babies

Babies delivered by Caesarean section with a total absence of labor miss the protracted contractions that accompany a normal delivery, and which stimulate the baby's peripheral nervous system and principal organs of survival. Consequently, these babies will benefit even more from a regular massage. As well as all the conventional benefits, a regular period of time spent massaging your baby also will give you the opportunity to strengthen your emotional attachments. Attempts at bonding may have been difficult at your baby's birth because of the medical attention required immediately after surgery and because your body needs time to recover, physical closeness can be made more difficult by your inability to lift and carry your baby while your body is healing.

Following a Caesarean section, you can use some of your recovery period to lay with your baby and introduce the massage routine for the very young baby (see pages 10–16). By the time your baby is ready to move onto a more formal routine, you should be more able to lift and carry him. Until your scar has healed, it is best not to do anything that puts pressure on your lower abdomen. Once you feel able to lift and carry your baby, keep your arms as close to your body as you can. Never try to lift him at arm's length, as this will place enormous strain on your lower back and belly. Caesarean babies can be more prone to lethargy, so massaging your baby will give him the stimulation that he needs, as well as the opportunity for you to check and promote his structural health and engage with him emotionally.

EXTRA BOOST
Massage can give a Caesarean baby the stimulation he needs to thrive.

Premature Babies

Given the high quality and sophistication of current neonatal care, most premature babies—including some weighing as little as 900 grams—survive. Some premature babies are fed intravenously and all have their heart rates, body temperatures and blood pressures constantly monitored within a sterile incubator. Because of these conditions, touching and stroking can be difficult, but you can still make contact with the most accessible parts of your baby's body, starting with his hands and feet.

Very premature babies can be hyper-sensitive to touch, but once they are a little more mature, their mother's touch is extremely beneficial. A baby who spends a long period of time in an incubator can associate touch with medical procedures and may cry when handled.

The staff in the special care baby unit will encourage you to touch your baby and—when and where possible—hold and handle him to engage in as much skin-to-skin contact as is possible.

Touching and stroking your baby will help him to thrive. Be patient—observe your baby and pay attention to his response.

At first, you could try just laying your relaxed hand or hands onto your baby's skin.

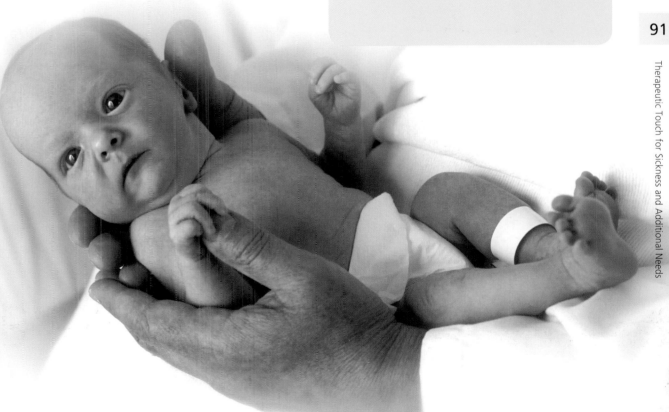

BENEFITS FOR PREM BABIES
Studies show that premature babies, if gently massaged for 15 minutes daily for ten days, absorb their food more easily and gain weight faster than those who are not massaged. Babies massaged in this way have been reported to have left the hospital six days earlier than babies who are not massaged.

Visual Impairments

Children with a visual impairment can benefit greatly from a regular massage. Perhaps even more than most babies, these children have a profound need for tactile stimulation. The sense of touch can provide a means of communication that allows the child to receive sensory information about her external world and a means to interact with it.

The impairment of one sense often leads to the greater development of another and this is especially true of touch. Children who are visually impaired depend upon their sense of touch to give form and recognition to the objects in their external world. Given regularly, massage can bring you more in touch with your child. This can make it easier for you to guide her towards the objects she will use in her everyday life. It will also help her to overcome any resistance she may have to being touched and encourage her to be more socially interactive.

When you introduce massage, it is important to do it slowly. Begin by stroking your baby gently—talk to her and be attentive to her response. One mother I knew would close her eyes when she massaged her child. She would talk and sing and maintain a wealth of physical contact—stroking, kissing and keeping her face very close to her baby's.

STIMULATING THE OTHER SENSES
To engage senses such as sound and smell, talk softly and keep your face close to your baby's as you massage.

Hearing Impairments

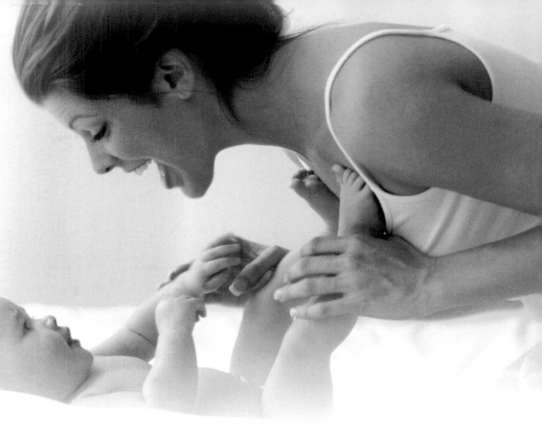

Babies with hearing impediments will benefit from massage. Given regularly, massage will encourage your baby's development and help you to appreciate the ways in which he communicates. This will strengthen your emotional relationship and add to your child's self-esteem. A baby who has a hearing impairment needs to be talked to and given lots of visual cues, as well as plenty of physical expressions of affection. Speak to your baby and mouth the words clearly as you say them, so that your baby can focus on you fully.

Introduce massage slowly and gently to overcome any initial tactile resistance. Stroke your baby and maintain eye contact as you explain what you are doing as you do it. Keep the massage enjoyable and pay close attention to your baby's response.

KEEP IN VOICE CONTACT
Talk to your baby as you massage him. Stay close and use lots of facial expressions of approval and affection.

Some babies with hearing or visual impairments are slow to crawl and walk. This may be because they are more resistant to lying on their bellies—they feel cut off from what is going on around them. So when you massage your baby's back, try laying him supported on a cushion from the waist up.

Talipes

This is a congenital deformity in a baby's foot or feet, which twists the foot out of shape or position. One of the most common forms of talipes is where the baby's foot turns inwards, often as a result of his position in the womb. This can be mild or severe and can sometimes be rectified by physiotherapy or if not, by a minor surgical procedure. To straighten the baby's foot, the heel must extend. For the heel to do so, the calf muscle must relax and stretch to allow the movement. Here are some massage techniques that you can use, but check with your physiotherapist before you begin, and show him or her what you plan to do.

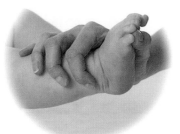

1 Kneeling comfortably on your feet on a cushion, pull your baby's lower leg and foot hand-over-hand through your palms. With your thumb turned downwards, draw your hand down your baby's calf. Follow through and turn the foot outwards to extend the heel as far as it will allow—without using any force.

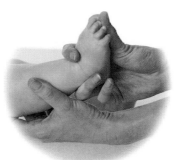

2 Hold the foot in this position while you massage your baby's calf with your other hand.

• **Continue for a few minutes or as long as your baby will allow. Repeat twice a day—morning and evening.**

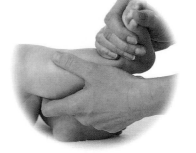

3 Now hold your baby's foot in the same position as you stroke and stimulate the muscle on the side of his shin with your fingertips.

4 Sitting comfortably with your back supported, raise your knees and let your baby squat on your belly with his back resting against your knees. His knees should be flexed and open with his feet resting against your chest or waist. Massage your baby's calf while simultaneously trying to extend the heel by pressing his foot against your chest or waist. Make sure you support him so that he cannot propel himself over your knees.

• **Continue for a few minutes or as long as your baby will allow. Repeat morning and night.**

Cerebral Palsy

This condition is attributed to a lack of development of the part of the brain concerned with movement and posture. Learning and visual difficulties including poor speech, hearing and vision may also be present if adjoining parts of the brain are also affected. The effects vary from child to child and range from slight to severe.

There are three recognized forms of cerebral palsy: ataxia—an unsteady walk with balancing difficulties; spasticity—disordered control of movement mostly associated with stiff muscles; and athetosis—uncontrollable or involuntary movements of different parts of the body. Children who are severely affected by cerebral palsy can require full-time care and postural support. On a day-to-day basis, massage can bring a moderate to high degree of relief and an improvement in the quality of their lives. If you are not already massaging your child, enlist the help of your physiotherapist and show him or her what you wish to do.

Any improvement in muscle tone brings with it more potential for movement and can influence posture. Massage can relieve the cramps that result from stiff muscles. Chronic wind and constipation often caused by poor posture and the lack of movement and mobility can be relieved. Circulation can be enhanced and a regular period of one-to-one physical contact through the medium of massage will also improve communication.

Cerebral palsy can go unrecognised for the first year or more, so if you have reason to believe that your child may be affected, seek medical advice. If your baby has been diagnosed as suffering from this condition, the sooner you begin to massage her, the better. Obviously, never try to force open or closed any of your baby's joints—modify the techniques to suit your baby. If your baby resists being naked, massage her clothed. Introduce the massage slowly—maybe one part of your baby's body at a time. You could start with her hands and feet, then her hands and arms, then her feet and legs, to build up a routine. Try to massage your baby daily and if you encounter any difficulties, consult your physiotherapist.

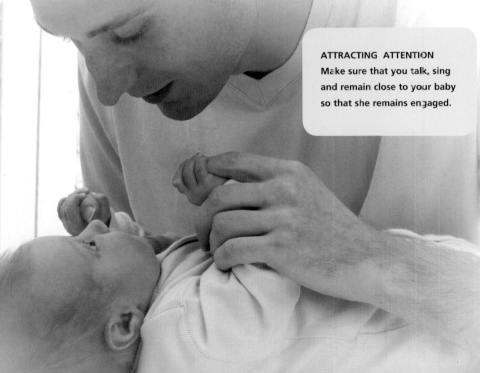

ATTRACTING ATTENTION
Make sure that you talk, sing and remain close to your baby so that she remains engaged.

95

Therapeutic Touch for Sickness and Additional Needs

Index and Acknowledgements

Acknowledgements

Thank you to all the mums, dads and babies who helped with the photography for this project.

Picture credits
Babyarchive.com p8, p22, p23
Photolibrary.com p61, p77, p90, p91, p92, p93